Examination of the Newborn

Doctors or midwives carry out an examination of all newborn infants within 24–48 hours of life. The purpose of the examination is to exclude major congenital abnormalities and reassure the parents that their baby is healthy. *Examination of the Newborn* provides a practical, step-by-step guide for midwives and other practitioners undertaking this role. It also encourages the reader to view each mother and baby as unique, taking into account their experiences preconceptually, antenatally and through childbirth. *Examination of the Newborn* covers:

- normal fetal development
- parents' concerns and how to respond to them
- the impact of antenatal diagnostic screening
- the events of labour and delivery
- the clinical examination of the neonate
- the identification and management of congenital abnormalities
- accountability and legal issues

The text is designed so that each chapter can be read independently and contains useful summaries and scenarios. *Examination of the Newborn* provides midwives and other practitioners concerned with neonatal examination with a comprehensive guide to the holistic examination of the newborn infant.

Helen Baston is a Lecturer in Midwifery and Researcher at the Mother and Infant Research Unit, University of Leeds.

Heather Durward is Staff Paediatrician at The Royal Hospital, Chesterfield.

Examination of the Newborn

A Practical Guide

Helen Baston and
Heather Durward

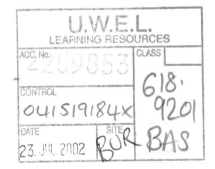

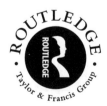

ROUTLEDGE
Taylor & Francis Group

LONDON AND NEW YORK

First published 2001
by Routledge
11 New Fetter Lane, London EC4P 4EE

Simultaneously published in the USA and
Canada
by Routledge
29 West 35th Street, New York, NY 10001

Reprinted 2002

*Routledge is an imprint of the Taylor & Francis
Group*

© 2001 Helen Baston and Heather Durward

Typeset in Janson and Futura by Prepress
Projects Ltd, Perth, Scotland

Printed and bound in Great Britain by
TJ International Ltd, Padstow, Cornwall

British Library Cataloguing in Publication Data
A catalogue record for this book is available
from the British Library
Baston, Helen, 1962–
    Examination of the Newborn: A Practical
    Guide/Helen Baston and Heather
    Durward
        p. cm.
Includes bibliographical references and
index.
ISBN 0–415–19184–X (hb) – ISBN 0-
415-19185-8 (pbk)
1. Infants (newborn) – Medical
examinations. I. Durward, Heather,
1960–.   II. Title.
[DNLM: 1. Physical Examination –
Infant, Newborn. WS 141 B327e 2000]
RJ255.5B37 2000
618.92′01–dc21 00-036621
CIP

For our husbands,
Simon and John,
and our beautiful children,
Hannah, Joseph and Sarah

Contents

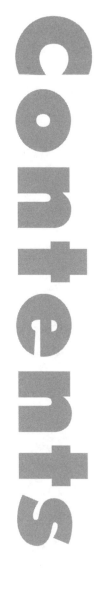

Figures

Tables

Preface

A comprehensive, clinical examination is performed on all babies, usually within the first 48 hours of life. It comprises a full physical assessment to reassure parents that their baby is healthy, fully developed and has no abnormalities. This clinical examination includes auscultation of the heart and lungs, detailed examination of the eye, palpation of the abdomen and assessment of the hips. It is performed in addition to the physical examination of the baby undertaken by midwives shortly after delivery of the baby.

Routine examination of the neonate is accepted as good practice (Hall 1996), and its value in terms of addressing parental concerns (Hall 1999) and providing parents with knowledge about what to expect from their baby (Walker 1999) is recognised. According to a large retrospective review of babies examined at 6–8 weeks of age (Gregory *et al.* 1999), the clinical examination detects only 44% of congenital defects of the heart (half of heart defects do not present at 1 day of age), but it remains the best opportunity for early detection. Neonatal examination also provides a vital opportunity for detecting congenitally displaced hips, which with early treatment results in complete resolution in most cases (Gerscovich 1997).

The examination provides a unique opportunity for the practitioner to promote health and instil confidence in the new family unit. For this to be accomplished, however, the examiner must be able to combine a sound understanding of the physical aspects of the examination with an awareness of the many other significant influences that affect the parents' perception of their baby. Parents also need to be treated as individuals; their need for reassurance will be based on their experiences of pregnancy and childbirth.

For the first time in one text, *Examination of the Newborn: A Practical Guide* brings together not only the clinical aspects of the examination but also the professional and legal frameworks that underpin this important screening event. It also encourages the practitioner to consider the woman and her family as unique, influenced by many factors, including social, economic and medical. This text does not replace the excellent sources of information found in individual chapters in larger texts but provides a valuable source of essential information within one compact volume. It will raise practitioners' awareness of the issues that relate to the first examination of the newborn and thus invoke a thirst for further reading of work referred to within the text.

As the length of postnatal hospital stay is declining, this first examination is often combined with the traditional discharge examination which confirms the baby's fitness to go home and thus places the care of the baby in the hands of the parent(s). Ramsay *et al.* (1997) in a study of 9,712 babies compared clinical outcomes in babies who had either one or two neonatal examinations. They concluded that there was no clinical difference in the detection and management of abnormalities between the two groups. As many maternity units have adopted this policy of one examination (irrespective of the length of hospital stay), it is important to ensure that the opportunity is not missed to provide advice and support for the new family unit.

Examination of the Newborn: A Practical Guide offers all practitioners involved in undertaking this clinical role with a comprehensive framework with guidance for safe, effective care. The examination of the newborn has traditionally been undertaken by paediatric senior house officers or general practitioners and now increasingly by midwives and neonatal nurses. The roles of the midwife and neonatal nurse are expanding within neonatal care. Further educational opportunities have enabled practitioners to develop enhanced clinical skills in accordance with the frameworks defined by their regulatory body, the United Kingdom Central Council (UKCC). Such role expansion has become increasingly valuable as practitioners strive to enhance the quality of services that they provide. For example, supported by the publication of the document *Changing Childbirth* (DOH 1993) midwives have explored ways that enable them to provide continuity of care to women and their families. One popular model is midwifery-led care, in which low-risk women are cared for by midwives who assume the role of lead professional. Medical support is only requested if a problem is identified.

This system, however, often falls down in the postnatal period. Although fit and healthy, postnatal women are often transferred into the community by midwives without medical input; this responsibility does not extend to the transfer of the baby. Thus, midwives are seeking to achieve competence to undertake the clinical examination of the neonate in order to provide a total package of care for low-risk women and their families.

The clinical examination of the newborn is also becoming an issue because of the increasing number of home deliveries. The majority of home births take place without medical cover, and general practitioners, who are not involved in intrapartum care, are sometimes unable to perform this examination. Women are sometimes faced with a request to take their baby to the hospital to be examined, despite a normal pregnancy and labour (Thorpe-Raghdo 1995). Many midwives feel that they are ideally placed to undertake this role after undergoing appropriate education and supervised clinical practice.

This education is now a reality. Experienced neonatal nurses and midwives are able to access specific programmes that combine theory with clinical practice. Such courses also provide the practitioner with the opportunity to look carefully at the role of the examination of the newborn infant and explore how it can be enhanced. It must be emphasised that the primary skill used by the practitioner when examining the neonate is the validation of normality. With increasing experience and knowledge, nursing and midwifery practitioners will be able to identify specific medical conditions; however, the *diagnosis* of abnormality remains the remit of the medical practitioner.

The First Examination of the Newborn: A Practical Guide takes the examination of the newborn into a new phase, taking a family-centred approach to this important consultation. This text encourages *all* practitioners with responsibility for the examination of the newborn to see each baby as being unique, an individual born into a complex community.

Examination of the Newborn: A Practical Guide is a particularly useful text. Although the chapters are related to each other, they are designed so that they can also be read independently.

Chapter 1 sets the scene for an individualised approach to the examination of the newborn baby. In order to do this the practitioner needs to consider preconceptual issues that affect women and how these may manifest during the examination of the baby. It alerts the examiner to the fact that each baby is the result of a unique combination of factors and that, through developing an appreciation of these, the examiner will be able to focus the examination to meet the specific needs of the family unit.

Chapter 2 considers normal fetal development in the light of the potential hazards to which the fetus may be exposed during its development. For the practitioner to be able to offer practical advice to women, an evidence-based approach to care is essential. This section provides a detailed look at the literature regarding the hazards to the fetus. It encourages the reader to develop strategies for answering the concerns voiced by parents during the examination.

Chapter 3 focuses on normal antenatal care and how fetal wellbeing is assessed. It highlights the dilemmas associated with antenatal diagnostic screening in order to provide the practitioner who examines the newborn with insight into the potential anxiety that may have been a dominant factor throughout the pregnancy.

Chapter 4 addresses some of the events that could occur during labour and delivery and could affect the health of the neonate. It also considers the implications of some of the choices that women make about how they would like their labour to be managed.

Chapter 5 takes the practitioner through the complete examination of the newborn, step by step, and focuses on the normal neonate.

Chapter 6 considers the most frequently encountered congenital abnormalities and describes their initial management.

Chapter 7 highlights the issues of accountability and medical negligence that are particularly important for the practitioner examining the newborn baby. It discusses the related aspects of care, such as informed consent and record keeping.

Examination of the Newborn: A Practical Guide provides a comprehensive guide to the holistic examination of the newborn. It provides the practitioner with a resource of related literature and concludes with an appendix of national support groups.

Acknowledgements

We would like to express our gratitude to our families and friends whose support and encouragement have made this book possible. The valuable contribution of colleagues from a variety of disciplines must also be acknowledged, in particular Stephen Swan and Lesley Daniels. Ian Pickering remains a constant source of inspiration in striving for excellence in the provision of all aspects of health care. We would like to express our gratitude to Keith R. Walton for his sensitive artistic contribution to the illustrations in this text.

We would like to thank all at Routledge for their guidance and our reviewers for their constructive comments.

Note to reader

For the sake of convenience, the feminine, third person pronoun will be used when referring to the practitioner, and masculine third person pronoun for the baby. This usage does not reflect any bias on behalf of the authors.

Chapter 1

In the beginning

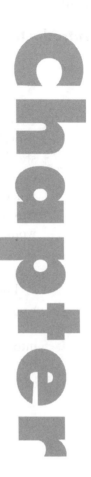

- Introduction
- Becoming a mother
- Premature and mature motherhood
- Infertility
- Questions that new parents may ask
- Summary

Introduction

The aim of this chapter is to set the scene for a comprehensive and sensitive examination of the newborn infant. Each woman's experience of becoming a mother is different and unique to her individual circumstances. The practitioner who examines her baby will be able to provide a woman-centred approach to this important examination if she does so with an appreciation of the factors that may influence the experience of motherhood. Such an understanding will also enable the practitioner to place in context any questions that may be raised by parents. Failure to consider the unique circumstances of individual women and their immediate families could potentially lead to care that is ritualistic. Parents should feel that the practitioner who examines their baby is focused specifically on them.

There are a multitude of variables that will impact on individual women and their experiences that we can only glimpse at in this context. This chapter provides a taster to help you reflect on how each journey into parenthood will be different and that this uniqueness must be reflected in the care that each woman receives. It aims, therefore, to encourage the practitioner to consider:

1 factors that may influence a woman's decision to start a family;
2 the implications of premature and mature motherhood;
3 the experience of women who have become pregnant through assisted conception; and
4 questions which new parents may raise.

Scenarios will be used to explore specific issues, focusing on the role of the practitioner undertaking the first examination of the newborn.

Becoming a mother

The decision to embark on the pleasure of parenthood is rarely made immediately prior to conception but is a culmination of a woman's culture, age, social class, peer pressure and relationship status. Each decision to 'try for a baby' is unique to that individual, and may or may not involve the prospective father. Indeed, it may not have been a conscious decision at all, but the result of lack of knowledge, limited access to effective contraception or a *laissez faire* approach to unprotected sexual intercourse. In the USA it is estimated that there are 3.5 million unplanned pregnancies each year (Klima 1998).

However, most pregnancies are planned and, according to Woollett (1991), having children is central to most women's identity. Not only does having a baby confer adult identity but also is an expression of womanhood, being female. It is almost like becoming part of a club where undergoing childbirth and the experience of bringing up a child are the essential prerequisites of membership. There is a common bond with other mothers, each having been through pregnancy, delivery and sleepless nights. Children also bring the security of a long-term relationship, and the decision to have children may even have been made because of loneliness in a marriage (Jennings 1995).

Occasionally, having a child may be part of a very specific long-term plan. For example, it is a consideration in some families, for example where there is a child with special needs, for parents to have more children than originally anticipated. This is not in an attempt to make up for the disability but to prevent a sibling with a handicapped brother or sister bearing the sole responsibility for their care when the parents are elderly or infirm.

For some women there is considerable pressure on them to reproduce because they are in a stable relationship or because they have reached a certain age. Such expectations may be part of a particular culture that may also dictate not only when parenthood should be considered but also the ideal family size and preferred gender of the children. Each cultural group also has norms and rituals associated with the birth of a new family member. It is essential that the practitioner becomes familiar with the particular customs that pertain to the client groups in her locality, so that they can be anticipated and accommodated with respect.

Premature and mature motherhood

Teenage pregnancy

Britain has the highest percentage of teenage mothers despite a fall in the number of live births to teenage girls in England and Wales, from 83,000 in 1971 to 45,000 in 1996 (Office for National Statistics 1998). Consequently this situation has been the target of successive government policy; hence teenagers are aware that their pregnancy may be viewed negatively by society. The practitioner examining the baby of a teenage mother will need to do so with an awareness of the attitudes that this young woman might already have encountered.

The probability of a teenage pregnancy occurring is increasing because the age of maturity and first sexual encounter is declining in females (Alcock 1992). There is a tendency for teenagers to think that it will not happen to them. In an Oxford study of 733 girls undergoing termination of pregnancy, more than 40% were not using any contraception at the time of conception (Duncan *et al.* 1990). Teenage pregnancy is often cyclical between generations and this has been illustrated in a study by Pheonix (1990), who found that in a group of 16- to 19-year-olds, 40% were the daughters of women who had also had their first babies before the age of 20.

Young mothers are often viewed with negative attitudes by both professionals and society. Having a baby below the age of 20 years has been linked with poor outcomes such as increased perinatal morbidity and welfare dependency (Jones *et al.* 1986). However, studies have also shown that if other factors are considered and accounted for, such as parity, the effect of maternal age on the outcome is greatly reduced (Butler *et al.* 1981). Other variables such as overcrowding and social class are more predictive of a poor perinatal outcome.

Teenage pregnancies are not always accidental but sometimes carefully planned. It may be a means of escaping an unhappy home (Roch *et al.* 1990), creating someone who will give them unconditional love (Alcock 1992), or a means of enhancing low self-esteem by achieving something of worth (Chaplin and McDiarmid 1992). It may also be the conscious decision of two committed individuals and should not be viewed as a childish error of judgement.

The young mother will undoubtedly have experienced negative attitudes towards her at some stage during her pregnancy. The practitioner examining her baby can help boost her confidence and morale by focusing on the positive aspects of her achievement. It is also an opportunity to raise issues such as immunisation or how to recognise when the baby is unwell as part of the natural flow of the examination, rather than in a preaching or superior manner.

Mature motherhood

The age at which women decide to commence child-rearing is increasing in developed countries; for example, in Britain the average age of mothers for all live births increased from 26.4 years in 1976 to 28.6 years in 1996 (Office for National Statistics 1998). A similar pattern is evident in the USA (Corson 1998). Some women postpone the onset of motherhood even longer, and this delay, it could be argued, may have both positive and negative sequelae.

Regarding the clinical aspect of pregnancy over the age of 35, many women in the past have been labelled 'high risk' and subject to extra obstetric care. A review of the literature (Katwijk and Peeters 1998) concludes that, providing the woman is in good health generally, there is no justification for extra antenatal care. However, an American study (Gilbert *et al.* 1999) found an increased rate of operative delivery (Caesarean section, forceps and suction) in nulliparous women over 40 years of age (61%) compared with women aged between 20 and 29 years (35%). Women who are over the age of 35 when they conceive have an increased risk of having a baby with Down's syndrome, and the issues surrounding antenatal screening for this condition are discussed in Chapter 3.

A woman who waits until she is older may feel emotionally and physically prepared for parenthood. If she is employed, she is more likely to have reached a more senior position within her chosen career and therefore be more financially secure. She may also have taken the opportunity to have accessed and implemented pre-conceptual advice, such as taking folic acid, reducing her alcohol intake and stopping smoking.

This rosy picture is idealistic and rather naive. Assuming that the woman is employed, she is more likely to feel socially isolated when she does give up work and be concerned that she is loosing her place on her chosen career ladder. If she has always been at work during the day she may have had little opportunity to develop close links and friendships with her neighbours. It may be difficult for her to combine motherhood with employment in the future because of shift patterns or inadequate child care facilities, and this may be a source of anxiety, especially if her wage was relied on. Particularly in areas of high male unemployment, many women are the sole wage earners, sometimes combining more than one job in order to pay the bills.

Women can face financial hardship at any age and may approach the practitioner who examines their baby for information regarding the benefits that they are entitled to. In such cases, women should be offered current, high-quality written information in addition to referral to the appropriate member of the multidisciplinary health care team.

Avoiding stereotypes

We have taken a glance at some of the issues that mothers may face depending on their age. It is important to explore how this knowledge might influence the care that you give when undertaking the first examination of the newborn. Consider the following scenario:

> You are caring for two women whose babies need their first neonatal examination before they go home from hospital. One mother is 15 and the other is 40 years of age. Before you undertake the examinations, you take a moment to reflect on the assumptions and stereotypes that you have of these women. How can you ensure that you provide appropriate care?

In order to illustrate the fact that professionals often categorise certain types of women, some of the common stereotypes that are attributed to teenage mothers are listed below. Of course, such descriptions could also be applied to the 40-year-old mother. The fact is that unless we know, we should not assume.

1 Limited knowledge regarding baby care: It is very easy to assume that because one mother is young that she has no experience caring for young babies. It could actually be the case that she has played a large part in the care of younger siblings and is confident and adept, and looking forward to caring for her own child.
2 Unplanned pregnancy: On the contrary, this may have been a much wanted and intended pregnancy
3 Unsupported, lonely and isolated: This young woman may have a very close network of friends and family who will be involved in the care and support of this new family. Many families make sacrifices to ensure that new babies have the latest equipment and clothes that they need.

Of course, in reality, all of the above descriptions of the teenage mother may have been applicable. In order to elucidate the facts about any new mother and therefore provide appropriate care, the practitioner should ask each mother the following questions:

- What experience does she have of young babies?
- How does she feel about the thought of taking the baby home?
- What support will she have in the first few days at home?
- Does she have any worries about caring for the baby?

These need not be direct questions, but part of the conversation between the mother and practitioner during the baby's examination.

We have considered how some women choose to delay motherhood; however, for some women this may have been involuntary. The baby that you examine may have taken many years of investigations or painful treatments to achieve.

Infertility

Childbearing has been described as a phase in the life cycle of the family, preceded by the 'couple phase' and followed by a number of new phases including 'toddler phase', and so on (Raphael-Leff 1991). It is therefore suggested that this is the usual course of events, the natural progression from finding security in a relationship. Childlessness has a negative image and often leads women to become stigmatised irrespective of whether or not it is a chosen status. Some women will therefore go to their physical, psychological and financial limits in order to become a mother.

The success rate for the many techniques that are used to treat infertile couples vary from centre to centre (Human Fertilisation and Embryology Authority 1999). Success is also influenced by factors such as the cause of infertility, age (particularly the age of the oocyte), sperm and embryo quality, previous obstetric history and pre-existing morbidity.

There is also inequality in the provision of treatment for infertility; many centres offer free treatment on the National Health Service; however, the access criteria vary widely along with the length of waiting lists, described in detail in the National Survey (National Infertility Awareness Campaign 1998). The result is that most couples pay for treatment, which may amount to thousands of pounds.

It may not be evident from examination of the woman's case notes whether or not she has undergone investigations or treatment for infertility, especially if donated gametes have been used and the couple wish to keep this a secret. This is entirely their right under the Human Fertilisation and Embryology Act 1990. The practitioner examining the baby must not assume, therefore, that the baby's parents are its biological ones (this may also apply if the baby has been delivered from a surrogate mother). If, however, the mother does disclose having received fertility treatment and this is recorded in her case notes, some of the abbreviations shown in Table 1.1 may be documented.

TABLE 1.1 Methods of assisted conception

Type	Description
IVF (*in vitro* fertilisation)	Collected eggs are mixed with semen in the laboratory for 48 hours. Only fertilised oocytes are replaced transcervically into the uterus
ICSI (intracytoplasmic sperm injection)	Prepared sperm injected directly into the oocyte in the laboratory and replaced into the uterus after 48 hours
GIFT (gamete intrafallopian transfer)	Oocytes are replaced with prepared sperm directly into the fallopian tube 36 hours after their recovery
Oocyte donation	Donor oocyte with partners prepared sperm
IUI (intrauterine insemination)	Seminal fluid deposited directly into the uterine cavity around the time of ovulation
DI (donor insemination)	Donor sperm used to fertilise maternal oocyte

After the birth, it is a possibility that the mother may feel quite detached or even indifferent to her new baby, despite her long wait. This is difficult for both her and her partner to cope with, especially when everyone else is so pleased and relieved at the successful outcome. Women will benefit from the gentle reassurance that this is a common reaction following childbirth, and that it sometimes takes time for mother and baby to form a strong bond. The literature does not support the hypothesis that parents of IVF children are maladaptive, although more empirical research in this area is required (McMahon *et al.* 1993).

> Consider your response to a parent who expresses concern about the effects of infertility treatment on the newborn baby.

The mother whose baby was conceived through the application of reproductive technology may have concerns about the effect of the drugs that she was given in order to maintain her pregnancy. Such worries are not entirely unfounded in view of the devastating effects of such drugs as diethylstilboestrol, which was used to prevent recurrent miscarriage and led to cases of genital cancer in babies exposed *in utero*, and thalidomide, which was used to treat nausea and vomiting in pregnancy and was held responsible for many severe limb defects. We await with trepidation any sequelae of assisted conception in either the mother or the fetus.

There is no evidence to suggest that babies born through IVF show a greater percentage of abnormalities than the general population. However, there is concern regarding children born through ICSI as there is greater manipulation of the oocyte. There is also the likelihood that male children may inherit their father's infertility problem. There are insufficient cohorts of children yet born through ICSI to support any final conclusions.

As the professional who examines the newborn infant it is impossible to predict or detect whether or not this baby will have an increased risk of morbidity in future life as a result of infertility treatment. It is possible, however, to state, should the parents inquire, that there is no current evidence to suggest that there will be major long-term effects from such treatment. In one study 100 babies who had been conceived *in vitro* were compared with babies conceived spontaneously (Fisch *et al.* 1997). There were no differences in the incidence of either major or minor abnormalities between these two groups of neonates. This was a small study and there is a need for much larger longitudinal studies before any concrete reassurance can be made. Increasingly, the embryos resulting from IVF will undergo pre-implantation diagnosis (PID), and thus their chromosomal status will be confirmed before being returned to the mother. However, it would be inappropriate to state categorically that this baby will not develop problems in the future (see Chapter 7).

Questions that new parents may ask

Having successfully given birth, the new mother will face many decisions and challenges ahead. She may turn to the practitioner for advice and guidance during this emotional time, and although you will not have all the answers it will be useful to consider some of the issues that could arise so that you can deal with them sensitively. The first thing you must ask yourself is: Am I the most appropriate person to answer this question?

This is particularly relevant if you are not the practitioner with continuing responsibility for that woman. In such circumstances, some questions, although you might have the knowledge to provide an answer, should be directed to the midwife who is assigned to the care of that woman. For issues such as breast feeding, for example, it may be the case that a variety of options have been tried or are planned. Without precise knowledge of previous discussions the practitioner may cause confusion. It may, however, be appropriate to give general advice about future care, but again her midwife should be informed of any concerns that may have been highlighted.

As you gain experience in the examination of babies, a pattern of frequent questions may emerge for your particular client group. Questions such as entitlement to benefits or the presence of local postnatal groups will need to be fielded with reference to the maternity services in your area. These are simple questions to answer, but some questions require more thought. There are a multitude of potential questions, but in order to help you consider the issues the new mother may face and how you as a practitioner might handle them, we shall explore one question in detail, that of employment.

Employment

For women who have achieved a successful career, it is can be difficult for them to fulfil the roles of both a full-time mother and a full-time worker. It has been suggested that it is almost impossible to combine these roles effectively because of the underinvestment in adequate child care provision. Many career opportunities are forgone in order to become a mother, confirming the stance that motherhood and paid employment are incompatible (Richardson 1993). There is often a conflict of interests: returning to work after the birth of a child enables the woman to develop her skills, communicate with other adults and be financially independent, but it also requires her to become 'superwoman' and juggle many responsibilities at the same time. Although many women are fortunate and share their commitments in a balanced relationship, many more do not and they often have to take time off work when the child is sick or to meet other, numerous responsibilities.

Women who, because of either financial necessity or personal choice, decide to return to work, no matter how definite that decision was, often suffer feelings of guilt. The new mother, overwhelmed by a myriad of emotions in the first few days after the birth, will be susceptible to the views and flippant statements of the professionals she meets.

Consider how a new mother might perceive the innocent questioning of the professional examining her baby when asked, 'do you work?'

The professional examining the baby may just be trying to make conversation spurred by the fact the parent's occupation was noted during close review of the case notes. Whether or not mothers should work is an extremely emotive issue. Many women simply do not have the choice and have to work in order to pay the bills. Others have chosen to stop working and stay at home while the children are young and they are able to 'happily relinquish ambition' (Hampshire 1984).

Many more women return to work on either a full- or part-time basis and will need support in order to minimise the associated guilt feeling they will inevitably experience. Even Hugh Jolly, an authority on aspects of childcare, states:

> Mothers should not feel guilty if they want to continue working while their children are still babies; it is better to be a happy 'part-time' parent than a depressed 'full-time' one.
>
> (1985: p. 136)

Of course, not everyone the new mother meets will express such enlightened views. Before the Second World War much attention was focused on the adverse effects on the institutionalisation of children and much of this work fuelled the theory of maternal separation and maternal instinct which became central to the work of Bowlby (1953). This considered opinion took the stance that it was indeed dangerous and stressful for children to be separated from their mothers and that mothers should not work but should stay at home caring for and nurturing their children. We now know that this is not the case and that as long as children have caring and consistent mother substitutes they will not come to any emotional harm (Hilton 1991). Despite this knowledge, it is often the former deprivation theory that remains deep seated in our culture and society. This means that not only do women feel guilty if they work, but also that family members, friends and colleagues have something to say on the matter (especially if they themselves stopped working after the birth of their children).

As with all these situations the converse is also true. Some women who do give up work are made to feel, by their career-minded acquaintances, that they are missing out on companionship, stimulation and, of course, money by staying at home. The role of the professional at these times of complex uncertainty and guilt is to be the neutral sounding board, enabling women to explore their own feelings without being judged or interrogated. At the end of the day, they will need to make a decision that is right for them, not for us.

> Consider how would you respond to a mother who asked you, 'when is the best time to return to work?'

This is a difficult question to answer and is of course linked to all the emotional guilt that relates to the previous scenario. There is, however, some useful ground that can be covered in response. For example, if the woman is breast feeding you can outline ways in which feeding can be maintained even after returning to full-time employment, and you can encourage her to seek the advice of the local feeding advisor, if there is one. In addition, there are many sources of further information such as community midwives, health visitors, La Leche League and the National Childbirth Trust (see Appendix 1).

It is useful to find out what plans she has and fill in any relevant details, such as 'yes, the baby might be sleeping through the night by then' or 'the baby will have had all injections by then', etc. Other useful suggestions might be to encourage her to take a day's annual leave each week for a while so that she becomes used to the new situation gradually. Health Visitors often know of local childminders that can be recommended or what facilities there are further afield. Whatever the woman is planning on doing it must be right for her, but she may ask you what you did when your children were young, if you have any. Even though there are certain stages at which it may be less traumatic for the mother to return to work, it will always be a source of anxiety and grief. This can be minimised by the professional who does not seek to impose rigid strategies but who listens to each individual and their unique social circumstances.

Some of the issues that face new parents have been considered along with the possible responses of the practitioner. No two women or their babies will be the same.

Consider this next account and reflect on how even women with very straightforward social and obstetric histories may face dilemmas when embarking on motherhood.

A personal account

I have always wanted children. When asked as a child what I wanted to be when I grew up, I would fervently retort, 'a mummy of course'. One might suppose that this was a consequence of my upbringing, the environment in which I grew up; however, this view point does not hold water when one considers my sister's reply to the same question, 'I'm going to be the Prime Minister'. I hope you don't think I am some sort of sissy or something, wanting to be a mummy for as long as I can remember, but it is the one thing in my life I never doubted for a second I could do. Even when my sister was undergoing investigations for infertility. Five years my senior, my sister was undergoing dye tests and hormone levels measurements when I was ready to start trying for our first baby.

I was in a dilemma. Should I wait until she became pregnant before I tried, because I did not want her to go through the added trauma of seeing me pregnant when she wanted to be? How long would it take? What if she could not have children – I'm sure she would not have wanted me to remain childless too. We decided to go ahead and try for our baby and I conceived straight away. My sister was the first to know and of course she was absolutely delighted, never once making me feel guilty. I never knew how she felt when we were not together.

We laugh now. Her daughter is the same age as my second child – she successfully conceived through IVF. She laughs at the many years of messing about with the whole range of contraceptives available, never knowing what a waste of time they were for her. I'm thankful I made the decision I did.

Summary

It is with appreciation of the preceding events, dilemmas and expectations that the practitioner examines the newborn infant. Although not all the information may be available, it is important not to jump to conclusions for they are likely to be inaccurate. This is difficult to avoid as everyone uses assumptions to help them interact with people they have never met (Green *et al.* 1990). However, generalisations apply to very few people, so it is more appropriate to verify details that are pertinent to the examination with the mother and use observational and listening skills to complement understanding of the wider context. The range of variables that influence the newborn's environment is vast and their combination covers an even greater range. They will all have an impact on the future life and opportunities of the newborn baby.

The next chapter will focus on normal fetal development, enabling the practitioner to relate the impact of intrauterine life on the examination of the newborn.

Chapter 2

Fetal development: influential factors

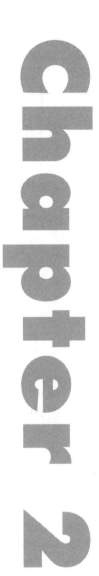

- Introduction
- Fetal development
- Summary

Introduction

Most pregnancies are free from complications, and the developing fetus grows strong and healthy in preparation for extra-uterine life. Some babies are, however, already compromised as a result of hazardous exposure during pregnancy. Before the practitioner begins the examination of the neonate, she will take the essential step of reading the mother's case notes and thus familiarising herself with the antenatal history. It will be in the light of this information that the baby is examined, and the practitioner will need to consider the implications of antenatal events for the mother and baby so that they can be anticipated. Some women may have spent months worrying about something that happened during the pregnancy and may look to the practitioner examining their baby for reassurance.

This chapter will begin with a brief account of normal fetal development to enable the reader to place in context the relevance of potential hazards, such as exposure to rubella during pregnancy. It will then discuss in more detail the major known antenatal risk factors, giving the practitioner a quick reference to their potential effects. Such knowledge will equip the reader with the ability to reassure and inform parents when they seek advice during the first examination of their baby.

Fetal development

It is important that the practitioner who examines the baby is able to apply knowledge of the stages of fetal development to the individual antenatal history of the baby under examination. Table 2.1 provides a guide to the development of the various systems of the body.

The gestational development of the fetus is extremely relevant to the examination of the newborn, especially if the woman has been worrying about a particular event in her pregnancy, such as an infection. If an abnormality is discovered, it is important to be aware that parents often blame themselves, and that they will make links with episodes from the antenatal period that might be causal in effect. Such concerns need to be listened to carefully and worked through systematically in order that they can be put in perspective and usually excluded.

The sections that follow will focus on the most relevant sources of potential fetal compromise and include smoking, alcohol, drug abuse, infection and environmental hazards. Information relating to fetal exposure to these influences is collected during the first consultation

Table 2.1 Development of fetal organs and systems

Organ/system	Development
Central nervous system	Spinal cord fusion process by 28 days after conception. Failure would result in neural tube defects
Peripheral nervous system	55 days after fertilisation
Digestive system	Stomach, small bowel, appendix, large bowel, rectum differentiated by 16 weeks. Development is so rapid that until 10 weeks' gestation it is accommodated within the uterine cavity. Failure to withdraw back into the abdominal cavity would result in either exomphalos or gastroschisis. Sucking and swallowing begin 8–12 weeks
Cardiovascular system	Primitive heart beating by 4 weeks after conception, valves and central septum of heart by 34 days
Respiratory system	Terminal bronchioles by 22 weeks' gestation. Surfactant-producing cells by 23–26 weeks
Urinary system	Producing and passing urine by 10 weeks
Genital system	Sex determined at fertilisation but may not be apparent until 12 weeks. In the male fetus the spermatogonia do not undergo first meiotic division until puberty, whereas in the female fetus this occurs between 8 and 16 weeks' gestation and the maximum number of primordial follicles has been achieved by 16–20 weeks
Eyes	Almost developed by week 13, although the eyelids remain fused until 24 weeks
Ears	Fully formed and functioning by 20 weeks, although the cartilage remains soft until 36 weeks
Limbs	By week 11 five fingers are distinguishable, and limb movements may also begin at this time. At 17 weeks nails can be identified. Bones begin to ossify at about 10 weeks' gestation
Face	Formed by 12 weeks. Clefts in the nose or palate occur when fusion of the maxillary processes is incomplete

between the woman and her midwife or doctor, the 'booking history', and recorded in her notes (see Table 5.1). Such data may then be updated throughout the antenatal period.

Smoking

Despite the wealth of information regarding the harmful effects on the fetus of smoking in pregnancy, approximately one in three women smoke at the beginning of their pregnancy (Madeley *et al.* 1989) and between 60% and 70% of those women continue to do so (USDHHS 1990). There may be many factors which contribute to this fact, including addiction to nicotine, habit, lack of support from family, friends and professionals or misconceptions regarding the effects of inhaling tobacco smoke. Approximately 4,000 fetuses are lost each year as a result of smoking in pregnancy (Royal College of Physicians 1993) and many more are harmed by the combined effects of carbon monoxide and nicotine.

Carbon monoxide	Found in cigarette smoke, it binds with haemoglobin, forming carboxyhaemoglobin. It is able to cross the placenta and thus reduces the oxygen-carrying capacity of both the mother's and the fetus's blood.
Nicotine	Causes generalised vasoconstriction, which leads to reduced blood flow to the uterus and is therefore another mechanism whereby the oxygen supply to the fetus is reduced.

In addition to the dangers that tobacco inhalation poses for all smokers (cancer, respiratory disease, cardiac disease) children exposed to cigarette smoke both before and after birth are also placed at risk of disease and even death. A summary of the major effects that smoking has on the mother and the fetus is shown in Table 2.2.

The practitioner has the ideal opportunity when examining the baby to offer advice and correct misinformation about this issue. It is, of course, important not to push information on women who are not expressing a desire to alter their smoking habits. However, failure to raise the issue may result in the women interpreting this as a professional being unsure of the facts (Haugland *et al.* 1996) or of not rating the effects of smoking in pregnancy and during their baby's developing

TABLE 2.2 A summary of the major effects of smoking on the fetus and mother

Effect	Reference
Low birth weight	Bardy *et al.* (1993): 1,237 pregnancies were studied, cotinine was discovered in 300 pregnancies and were classified as 'exposed'. After correction for parity, gender and gestational age the exposed newborns were, on average, 188 g lighter than non-exposed babies. See also Myhra *et al.* (1992), USDHHS (1990), Chattingius and Haglund (1997)
Increased incidence of glue ear	Strachan D. P. and Cook D. G. (1998): a quantitative systematic review of evidence relating parental smoking to acute and chronic otitis media. See also Gillies and Wakefield (1993)
Increased fetal, neonatal and perinatal mortality rates	Haglund B. and Chattingius S. (1990): a prospective study of 279,938 Swedish births reported that smoking doubled the risk of sudden infant death syndrome and a dose–response relation was noted. See also Butler *et al.* (1972), USDHHS (1990)
Increased risk of asthma	Weitzman *et al.* (1990): a retrospective examination of information relating to 4,331 children concluded that maternal smoking is associated with higher rates of asthma and an earlier onset of the disease. See also Neuspiel *et al.* (1989)
Reduced milk supply (mother)	Vio *et al.* (1991): ten smoking and ten non-smoking mothers' supplies of breast milk were compared and non-smokers were found to have significantly greater breast milk volume

years as a cause for concern. It is much more helpful to focus on the benefits of smoking cessation for the woman rather than being judgmental or adopting a moralistic tone.

Simply providing information alone, however, has been evaluated as being ineffective in persuading people to stop smoking (Campion *et al.* 1994). Information should therefore be given in addition to, not instead of, practical support and personal contact with trained professionals, a strategy which has been shown to be more effective (Walsh 1997). It is therefore important that the practitioner examining the baby is aware of local support groups and initiatives that the woman and her family can access.

It could be argued that, even if women do not make any changes as a result of information they receive, they still have a right to that information in order to make an informed choice about their health behaviour.

A useful model of change, developed by Prochaska and DiClemente (1983), identifies six possible stages that the individual might go through when considering stopping smoking. These are pre-contemplation, contemplation, preparation, action, maintenance and relapse. It is suggested that individuals need to go through each stage of the process in order to achieve successful 'maintenance', and that even if relapse into smoking occurs repeatedly, each time they attempt to quit smoking they are more likely to succeed. The practitioner examining the newborn baby can reassure a mother who expresses concern at having already relapsed that this happens to most smokers attempting to stop, but that they are now one step nearer to becoming a non-smoker in the future.

Even if the woman is a non-smoker it is important to discuss the risks associated with passive smoking for there may be family members who need a subtle reminder not to smoke in the same room as the baby. A study by Geary *et al.* (1997) demonstrated that over 50% of women did not receive information with respect to passive smoking. Many women are grateful for the extra ammunition to their request that visitors do not smoke near their baby by being able to say, 'they said at the hospital that babies who live in smoky environments are at increased risk of chest infections or even cot death', which is much more effective than saying, 'I'd rather you didn't.'

It is also important to note that almost a quarter of pregnant smokers do not declare this fact, and those who do frequently underestimate the number of cigarettes they smoke each day (Ford *et al.* 1997).

Consider the following scenario, where the practitioner examining the newborn baby has an ideal opportunity to correct misinformation:

> I was told that my baby would be small if I continued to smoke during my pregnancy, but he is bigger than my friend's baby, and she never smoked.

You may think that there is little point in discussing smoking issues with a mother who already has her 4-kg baby safely delivered. However, if she raises the issue, it is an opportunity to find out what she knows about the effects of smoking on children. The size of the baby is not always the most helpful argument for health professionals to use, as women can always quote examples similar to the above scenario. The fact is that babies of women who smoke will be on average 200 g lighter than babies whose mothers did not smoke (USDHHS 1990) and 10 mm shorter (Bardy *et al.* 1993) – not attributes that most parents would wish to be responsible for.

The woman in the above scenario is letting you know that she is a smoker, and it is therefore appropriate that you inform her of the risks associated with passive smoking, giving her practical advice in a non-judgmental way. It would be inappropriate to be prescriptive and make paternalistic statements about her smoking behaviour. She needs to know that if she made the decision to try to stop smoking that there are many resources available to her, but that in the mean time to smoke outside or in a separate room from the baby would be a positive step that she can take now. You could plant the seed that perhaps as the child grows up she might not want it to copy her role model as a smoker. The key is not to force further information on her but to take your queues from how receptive she is to each aspect.

Alcohol

In 1997 the Royal College of Obstetricians issued a press release which stated that there are no proven adverse effects on pregnancy outcome when women consume less than 15 units of alcohol per week during pregnancy. Florey *et al.* (1992) put the safe level at less than 10 units of alcohol per week. The fact is that there has been and will continue to be much controversy and debate over establishing what is a safe level of alcohol consumption.

It is known, however, that a moderate consumption of alcohol is linked with a reduction in birth weight and that a consistently high consumption of alcohol is linked with a series of characteristics that together are known as fetal alcohol syndrome (FAS). This syndrome was first described by Jones and Smith in 1973.

FAS affects 1 in 600 live births and is the third most common cause of mental retardation (Seidel *et al.* 1997). It comprises some or all of the following clinical features:

microcephaly
small eyes
hearing disorders
large ears
shallow philtrum
intrauterine growth retardation
thin upper lip
congenital abnormalities, such as cleft lip/palate, heart defects,
mental retardation

Affected babies may show signs of alcohol withdrawal at birth and therefore be irritable, jittery, have feeding problems and elicit a high-pitched cry. Babies demonstrating such symptoms should therefore be meticulously examined to exclude conditions such as atrial and ventricular septal defects and should be referred to a paediatrician for assessment.

There is evidence that alcohol is most teratogenic during organogenesis and development of the nervous system (see Table 2.1) (Armant and Saunders 1996). Kaufman (1997) describes how exposure to alcohol can induce chromosome segregation errors in the ovulated oocyte. Such eggs are unlikely to be fertilised but those that are either result in early miscarriage or, very rarely, proceed to develop into children with severe mental retardation. Alcohol consumption has been associated with reduced fertility in women (Jensen *et al.* 1998)

Consider the following expression of concern from a new mum:

> I'm really worried. I became pregnant after getting drunk at a party. I don't normally drink but I'm worried I may have harmed the baby.

The research states that for someone who is well nourished and is not a heavy drinker normally getting drunk in early pregnancy is unlikely to have caused the baby any problems (Tolo and Little 1993). It would be particularly valuable to explain to her the sort of problems associated with excessive alcohol consumption during pregnancy and systematically show her, for example, that the baby's head is the expected size, that its eyes, ears and lips all appear to be normal. Of course, you cannot tell her that her baby will not develop problems in the future, but that at the moment you do not have any concerns about the baby. If it is appropriate, you could perhaps make sure that she is aware of the potential danger of suffocation if she has the baby in bed with her after she has consumed alcohol, especially if, as new parents often are, she is extremely tired. Unsafe sleeping conditions are often implicated in cases of unexpected deaths in infants (Beal and Byard 1995), and the examination of the newborn is an ideal opportunity to inform *all* parents about current perspectives regarding safe sleeping conditions for babies (see Appendix 2)

Drug abuse

In cases where it is clearly evident from the woman's case notes that she has been abusing drugs during her pregnancy, the baby must be referred to a paediatrician in order that the need for medical treatment or long-term care can be assessed. However, not all women disclose their addiction.

The practitioner examining the newborn baby may be alerted to the possibility that the mother has abused drugs during her pregnancy if the baby demonstrates symptoms of withdrawal, including irritability, poor feeding, vomiting, high-pitched cry and tremor. The degree of withdrawal is dependent on the type of drugs and the amount consumed.

Heroin

High doses of heroin taken by the mother are likely to cause the baby severe problems in the perinatal period. The baby will demonstrate the symptoms of withdrawal mentioned above and is also more likely to be of low birth weight (Alroomi 1988). It is important to raise the issue that babies whose mothers are heroin addicts should not be given naloxone at delivery, as this could precipitate severe withdrawal. Therefore, for babies exhibiting symptoms of withdrawal, administration of naloxone at delivery should be excluded as a precipitating factor.

Researchers have had difficulty identifying the particular effects of heroin abuse because it is invariably used in conjunction with tobacco and alcohol, and the mother often has a poor nutritional status; these are factors which are known to have negative sequelae for the unborn child.

As the number of women who abuse drugs in pregnancy rises, the expertise of the agencies caring for them also increases. In areas where substance misuse is particularly prevalent, teams of professionals work together to offer support and treatment for pregnant women (Siney 1994, Hepburn 1993). The baby born to a mother on a low-dose methadone programme may not exhibit any symptoms at all or may have mild symptoms that persist for a few months (Roberton 1996).

A baby that is showing symptoms of opiate withdrawal should be referred to a paediatrician for management of care as long-term follow-up may be indicated. It should be nursed in a quiet environment and be offered small, frequent feeds.

Cocaine

Use of this central nervous system stimulant in pregnancy is linked with, shorter body length, reduced head circumference and intrauterine growth retardation associated with placental and uterine vaso-constriction (Polin and Fox 1998). Such effects may be confounded by the fact that cocaine is an appetite suppressant; hence its users are often of a poor nutritional status (McNamara 1995). The neonate, although not displaying consistent withdrawal patterns, is likely to be irritable and should therefore be nursed in a calm environment (Nora 1990).

Amphetamines

Plessinger (1998) describes the risks of adverse outcomes for the fetus exposed to amphetamines and mathampetamines. These include fetal growth retardation and cardiac anomalies, findings that have been confirmed in animal studies.

Cannabis

In a meta-analysis of over 32,000 women, English *et al.* (1997) concluded that in the amounts typically consumed by pregnant women cannabis does not cause low birth weight. Unlike many other forms of drug abuse, it has not been linked with an increased risk of perinatal mortality (Zuckerman *et al.* 1989). It has been suggested, however, that when cannabis is used with other substances, such as alcohol and tobacco in pregnancy, it can increase the negative consequences for the developing baby (McNamara 1995)

A note on breast feeding

For practical purposes it should be estimated that approximately one-tenth of the mother's drug intake will be delivered to the baby through the breast milk (Hull and Johnston 1993). It is important, therefore, that the benefits of breast feeding are carefully considered in the light of the possible harmful effects of drug use, and that the parents are given this information in such a way that they can make an informed decision.

Transplacental infection

Rubella

If a pregnant woman is exposed to primary rubella infection, especially in the first trimester, the baby may be born with one or a number of serious clinical features, including deafness, retinopathy, encephalopathy, deafness or a heart defect. The risk of congenital abnormality is greatest if the fetus is exposed to infection during the first 8 weeks of pregnancy, and this is evident in 85% of such babies (Hull and Johnston 1993). The risk gradually reduces with increasing gestation and is negligible after 22 weeks of pregnancy.

Toxoplasmosis

Toxoplasmosis is a parasitic infection caught from cat faeces and contaminated soil, raw or inadequately cooked meet and unpasteurised goats' milk products. It is thought that about half of the population will have been infected without realising it. If toxoplasmosis is contracted during pregnancy the risk of transplacental transmission is about four out of ten. Infection is most significant in early pregnancy but may affect the fetus at any stage. If maternal infection is confirmed during pregnancy, antibiotic therapy can reduce the risk of the fetus becoming infected. Infection could result in blindness or encephalopathy at birth, or the development of chorioretinitis in later life.

The practitioner examining the baby exposed to toxoplasmosis *in utero*, must refer it to a paediatrician for follow-up care.

Chicken pox

Chicken pox is caused by the herpes varicella zoster virus (HZV). Maternal primary infection in early pregnancy may lead to serious fetal anomalies (congenital varicella syndrome), including central nervous system damage and eye deformities, although these are rare. Neonatal morbidity is highest when the mother develops the rash in the week surrounding the birth, and it is associated with a mortality rate of approximately 30% (ACOG 1993). Babies born to infectious mothers should be referred to a paediatrician for possible treatment with acyclovir and/or vaccination.

HIV infection

There is no way of testing whether babies of HIV-infected mothers will ultimately develop the virus, for all such babies will have acquired antibodies via the placenta. It is only through long-term follow-up that HIV infection can be ruled out, and it is therefore important that such babies receive paediatric follow-up. Approximately one-third of babies will become infected, although infection cannot be diagnosed until the infant is 18 months old as maternal antibodies may persist until then. Breast feeding is contraindicated in the developed world, where the risk of transmission outweighs the benefits.

Cytomegalovirus (CMV)

CMV is the most common intrauterine infection, occurring in 0.4–2.4% of all live births (Seidel *et al.* 1997). The virus persists after primary infection and can be reactivated. It is estimated that between 1% and 5% of pregnant women become infected, with approximately 50% of those pregnancies being affected by the virus. A wide range of malformations may be caused, including microcephaly, growth retardation and nerve deafness, but only 5% will have clinical signs at birth. If infection is confirmed during pregnancy, audiology follow-up may be indicated.

Listeria

The source of the bacteria responsible for this bacterial infection is soft cheeses, unpasteurised milk products and meat products requiring reheating. It may be acquired by the fetus via the placenta or during delivery. Those infants infected before birth usually present with symptoms of septicaemia soon after delivery, and the associated mortality rate is approximately 30%. However, where maternal infection is confirmed, antibiotic therapy may improve the outlook for the fetus. Offensive liquor and placental abscesses may have been noted at the delivery. Infants becoming infected after delivery often present with meningitis (Seidel *et al.* 1997) and have a better prognosis.

Congenital parvovirus B19

This virus when contracted by the mother may lead to spontaneous abortion or hydrops fetalis in about 1% of those pregnancies that progress. Most maternal infections with this virus do not affect the developing fetus.

Environmental influences

Much has been published regarding the harmful effects of various substances that women may be exposed to in pregnancy (Foresight 1996). These range from the organophosphates present in pesticides to the lead in exhaust fumes. The effects on the developing fetus include congenital malformations such as cleft lip and hydrocephaly. World attention has also focused on the immediate and long-term effects of radiation after the Chernobyl disaster, including psychophysical effects (Nyagu *et al.* 1998).

However, it is almost impossible to attribute an abnormality to a particular cause. It is not always helpful to identify a source of the problem if an individual is powerless to do anything about it, such as car pollution. If the practitioner examining the newborn baby is asked to answer concerns about antenatal exposure to environmental hazards during pregnancy, the following the two examples can be used.

Anaesthetic gases

Anaesthetic gases increased the risk of spontaneous abortion before the introduction of scavenging (the system for the removal of waste gases), according to a meta-analysis (Boivin 1997). Hemminki *et al.* (1985) reported that there was no association found between anaesthetic gases and abortion and malformation, but they did report an association between exposure to cytostatic drugs and the incidence of malformations.

Electromagnetic field

A study conducted by Sorahan *et al.* (1999) sought information on the occupation of mothers of 15,041 children who had died of cancer in Great Britain between 1953 and 1981. It concluded that maternal occupational exposure to electromagnetic fields was not a risk factor.

Diet

We have already considered the potentially harmful effects of eating particular foods during pregnancy in terms of the risk of contracting such infections as listeria and toxoplasmosis. It is also suggested that there are risks to the fetus associated with the consumption of a diet that is nutritionally poor, for example low birth weight (Luke 1994). By the time the practitioner examines the newborn baby, it will already have been exposed to its mothers diet. Other than recognising a growth-retarded baby or the cherubic features of a baby that has been exposed to a high blood glucose level (see Chapter 6), it might be assumed that there is little need for the examiner to be conversant with dietary influences on fetal development. This is not so. It has been seen how opportunities exist during the examination of the newborn infant to correct misinformation and offer advice where appropriate. Consider the following scenario:

> My friend advised me to take folic acid before I got pregnant but I didn't like the idea of taking drugs during my pregnancy...well you hear of such awful things happening to babies because their mums took drugs, don't you? Anyway he's all right, isn't he?

There are a few misconceptions demonstrated here. Folic acid (0.4 mg daily) taken preconceptually and up until the twelfth week of pregnancy has been shown to reduce the incidence of neural tube defects by approximately 75% (Medical Research Council Vitamin Study Research Group 1991). This can be put into a realistic figure for parents by explaining that approximately two babies are conceived every day in England and Wales with this condition (Health Education Authority 1996). Therefore, if each woman planning a pregnancy took folic acid this could prevent 10 babies a week being born with this disabling abnormality. The fact that she has had a baby that is not affected with a neural tube defect does not mean that she is not at risk. Neural tube defects can develop in babies of women of any age and taking folic acid can reduce the risk of this happening. Folic acid has been tested very carefully and widely used by pregnant women and has not been associated with adverse effects on the developing baby.

Folic acid is inexpensive to purchase and is available on prescription from many family doctors. It may be useful to add that, when explaining to women how to reduce the risks of fetal abnormality, we often do not know what causes defects to develop. Therefore, when we do know of a course of action that can reduce the risk, we should consider it very carefully. Many women feel terribly guilty and blame themselves if their baby has an abnormality and this is exacerbated when there *might* have been a known preventative course of action.

The prevention of neural tube defects is just one example of how the practitioner can respond positively to women's comments and questions during their baby's examination. Verbal advice, especially when it applies to future decisions or lifestyle changes, should be followed by the appropriate literature.

> Follow your spoken word with written information.
>
> Find out what your local resources are.

Summary

It has been shown that the practitioner will need a thorough knowledge of a wide range of issues in order to be optimally equipped to undertake the first examination of the newborn. Although a comprehensive understanding of the physical aspects of the examination are essential, an ability to answer women's questions effectively is also crucial and has the potential to contribute to the long-term wellbeing of the family.

When there is evidence or even the suspicion that the mother has a history of alcohol or drug abuse, the practitioner examining the baby must ensure that the relevant support agencies are involved in the care and long-term support of this vulnerable family unit. Children growing up within this environment are more likely to suffer from physical and emotional neglect, the aetiology of which is complex and beyond the scope of this text. The mother's addiction may be a symptom of abuse that she herself is being or has been subject to and should not therefore be considered in isolation (McFarlane *et al.* 1996).

Chapter 3

Assessment of fetal wellbeing

- Introduction
- Antenatal care
- Summary

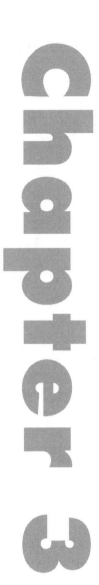

Introduction

The majority of pregnancies have perfect outcomes despite exposure to potential hazards along the way. However, one baby in 50 will have an abnormality at birth (Myles 1999), ranging from an extra digit to a major heart defect. The proportion of babies being born with abnormalities has reduced considerably in recent years. There are many possible reasons for this, including an increased awareness of the many potential risks that babies can be exposed to *in utero*, enabling some to be avoided. In addition, recent advances, such as the ability to discover the genetic profile of the fetus and to visualise the fetus as it is developing, enable parents to make decisions regarding therapeutic abortion if an abnormality is detected.

The general purpose of antenatal care is to:

1 monitor the health of the mother and baby;
2 educate on health and prepare for the future; and
3 screen for particular abnormalities.

It could be argued that examination of the newborn is a continuation of this process. It is therefore essential that the practitioner has a clear understanding of the events that have preceded the examination of the neonate.

This chapter will build on the previous chapters, focusing on how fetal wellbeing is monitored in the antenatal period. It begins with an overview of antenatal care and the importance of the 'booking history'. Particular emphasis is placed on antenatal screening and how that should be followed through when the practitioner examines the baby.

Antenatal care

The majority of antenatal care takes place in the community with the low-risk woman only going to hospital for ultrasonography at the beginning of her pregnancy or to see a doctor if she goes beyond her expected date of delivery. The woman who has a positive pregnancy test will usually make an appointment with either her family doctor (GP) or her community midwife. This first visit is an opportunity for the management of the pregnancy to be discussed and often features little in the way of clinical examination, although this will vary between individual practitioners. A hospital referral is usually made at this point, although the place of delivery should be chosen after a full discussion of all the available options (Department of Health 1993).

The booking history

This is probably the most important encounter that the woman makes with her community midwife in the whole pregnancy. Not only is it an opportunity to provide the woman with important information regarding diet, smoking and screening tests, but it also forms the basis of a relationship which will continue after the birth of the baby.

The booking history usually takes place in the community, at approximately 8–12 weeks of pregnancy. It comprises family history, medical history, obstetric history, social history, screening test counselling, antenatal examination and health promotion advice. This information is essential for the examination of the neonate and should therefore be carefully read by the practitioner before seeing the baby.

An attempt to examine a baby without any prior knowledge of antenatal events would be like applying a generic screening test without identifying the individual needs of the parents and baby. Of course, it would be possible to examine a baby clinically by going step-by-step through the procedure (see Chapter 5); however, a valuable opportunity to provide client-centred care would be missed. Knowledge of the history of a pregnancy should therefore be seen as essential, not optional. For examples of what the practitioner examining the baby should look for in maternal notes see Table 5.1.

Knowledge of the antenatal history can inform and enrich the examination of the baby. Consider the following scenario:

A mother, aged 40 years, decided to have an amniocentesis when she was 16 weeks pregnant because she was informed at her booking history that she had a 1 in 100 risk of carrying a baby with Down's syndrome. She had spent several days agonising over whether or not to have the test as she had taken 2 years to conceive and did not want to put her baby at risk. Having decided to have the test she then faced the prospect of waiting 3 weeks for the results. However, the cells taken from her amniotic fluid failed to culture and she was asked if she wanted to repeat the test. She declined on the basis that she could not put her baby at risk again and, also, by this time she had felt the baby move and had seen it several times during ultrasound scans. She therefore spent the rest of her pregnancy wondering if she had made the right decision and hardly daring to hope that her baby would be 'normal'.

The practitioner examining this baby, in the light of the knowledge about the amniocentesis, would be able to take deliberate steps to take the parents carefully through the examination of their baby, explaining exactly how Down's syndrome is identified clinically. This would be appropriate in view of the concerns and anxieties that they had experienced antenatally. Although the same clinical features would have been considered in the examination of a baby of a 25-year-old woman with no family history of Down's syndrome, it would not have been appropriate to overtly demonstrate this aspect of the examination.

It can be seen that prior knowledge of the antenatal history can enable the practitioner to enhance the parents' experience of their baby's examination. However, the practitioner must not be complacent. What may be regarded as a near perfect environment for fetal development, in terms of minimal known risk factors and an uneventful antenatal period, has the potential to result in an unexpected abnormality in the neonate. The practitioner should therefore *anticipate the probable and expect the unexpected*.

Despite the widespread use of antenatal diagnostic screening for fetal abnormality, most women worry that there might be something wrong with their baby. This has been found to be highest at the beginning and towards the end of the pregnancy and is prevalent in 90% of women (Statham *et al.* 1997). The first examination of the newborn is therefore a milestone whereby this fear of abnormality can either be dissipated or, in some cases, sensitively confirmed.

Antenatal screening tests

It is at the booking visit that all women, regardless of their previous medical or family history, are asked to consider the various tests that are available to them. For some women and their partners the decisions are straightforward. For others, however, this may be the first time that they have even considered the possibility that their developing baby is less than perfect. This could be the first step along a rocky road for the small proportion of women whose test results are not what they hoped for, and it is important that the practitioner who examines the baby once it is born is sensitive to the journey already travelled.

Questions may arise at the first examination of a newborn that require a thorough knowledge of the current research evidence, for example:

> I needed to have lots of scans in my pregnancy because I had a low-lying placenta. Do you think that this could have been harmful to my baby?

or you may need to show that you understand how test results are interpreted and the action that might follow:

> My triple test showed that I had a high risk of having a baby with Down's syndrome, but after lots of thought we decided not to have an amniocentesis. Does the baby look normal?

There is increasing evidence that antenatal screening for abnormality provokes anxiety. In a study conducted in Denmark (Jorgensen 1995) women undergoing alpha-fetoprotein (AFP) testing with false-positive results were interviewed at approximately 30 weeks' gestation. Forty-six per cent (56/123) of women whose results were reclassified as normal following an ultrasound scan described being severely anxious, and for some this anxiety was still present when completing the questionnaire.

Such studies highlight the need for the professionals who counsel women prior to screening to be provided with clear, realistic and unbiased information. Research funded by the Research Council (Smith *et al.* 1994) examined women's knowledge about aspects of screening for Down's syndrome. It involved 353 pregnant women and found, for example, that only 13% were aware that 5% of women were called back for further tests, and that only 32% knew that most women with positive results have normal babies. It is not surprising therefore that false-positive results contribute to antenatal anxiety. This may manifest itself in a barrage of questions for the professional undertaking the first examination of the newborn.

The following section will consider the main antenatal screening tests currently available. It must be appreciated that not all maternity units will offer the whole range of tests described.

Down's risk screening

Until the early 1990s only women over the age of 35 years were offered screening for Down's syndrome as its incidence is seen to rise dramatically with age. For example, the incidence of Down's syndrome at age 25 years is 1 in 1352 live births, rising to 1 in 167 at age 38 and being as high as 1 in 30 at age 44 (Rogers 1997).

However, over 70% of babies with Down's syndrome are conceived to mothers who are below 37 years of age. There are various tests available to women designed either to diagnose or assign the risk of a Down's syndrome pregnancy, including chorionic villus sampling (CVS), amniocentesis and maternal serum screening (triple test, double test or Bart's test)

Chorionic villus sampling

Chorionic villus sampling is a screening test that is available in many obstetric units. It involves the removal of a small sample of villi from the chorion frondosum, either transcervically or through the abdomen, and may be conducted in the first trimester of pregnancy.

It has an associated risk of miscarriage rate of up to 8.2 per 100, although, as Green and Staham (1993) note, this rate varies depending on maternal age, skill of the operator and reporting bias. This high risk of pregnancy loss is a high price to pay for the benefits of early diagnosis, but it is an extremely valuable test for couples with a family history of genetic abnormality, or for women who are sure that they could not possibly care for a child with a disability or life-threatening illness. Since actual tissue is biopsied, results are potentially available within 24 hours of the sample being taken (compared with 3 weeks for amniocentesis).

Ultrasound scanning in pregnancy

Ultrasound in pregnancy is an accepted and much valued part of pregnancy for the majority of women. It is viewed as a routine procedure, during which the baby is measured and after which a picture is obtained. However, it is seldom presented as the screening test that it is. In a study conducted by Crang-Svalenius et al. (1996), it was concluded that very few women were given information regarding the aims of a second trimester ultrasound scan, and fewer than half could not recall being told that there was a possibility that abnormality could be detected. Smith and Marteau (1995) found that the information that parents received regarding their routine anomaly scan was scant and was less than that received for the maternal serum screening.

Alternatively, many parents assume that because they have had an ultrasound scan in pregnancy and that nothing abnormal was detected, it can be concluded that the baby must be normal. Unfortunately, this is not the case. The sensitivity of the scan will vary according to the gestation at which it was performed, the skill of the ultrasonographer, the position of the fetus and the resolution of the equipment. In a study conducted by Leslie *et al.* (1996) the case notes were examined of mothers whose fetuses had potentially scan-detectable heart defects, i.e. other than patent ductus arteriosis or atrial septal defect, and only 38% had been diagnosed.

Ultrasound is also used to determine gestation, which is crucial for the interpretation of many antenatal screening tests, and it is more accurate than relying on dates alone (Wald *et al.* 1992). The number of ultrasound scans that women have varies considerably, and in England averages at over three per live birth (Robinson 2000). For some women, especially those who have had repeated scans during their pregnancy, the fact that their baby was exposed to ultrasound *in utero* will be a source of concern. Consider the following question, which the practitioner examining the newborn infant may be asked:

> I needed to have a lot of scans in my pregnancy because I had a low-lying placenta. Do you think this could have been harmful to my baby?

In responding to such anxieties, the practitioner must present a balanced answer. Parents need to be informed that there is no evidence to suggest that there is any harmful effect from the use of ultrasound in pregnancy, although it has been reported that there may be a link between ultrasound exposure and non-right-handedness, especially in boys (Salvesen and Eik-nes 1999). School performance at age 8–9 years has not been demonstrated to be altered by ultrasound exposure (Salvesen *et al.* 1992). The clinical usefulness of ultrasound must be balanced against the potential, as yet unqualified, risks. Although harmful effects have not been shown, the use of higher intensity ultrasound is increasing and it should continue to be monitored carefully.

As the expertise and experience of the technicians using ultrasonography increases, more markers suggestive of abnormality are being identified. Markers may occur in isolation or in association with other suspicious findings and include choroid plexus cysts, nuchal translucency, dilated renal pelvis (pyelectasia).

CHOROID PLEXUS CYSTS

These are relatively common and are identified in approximately 1% of fetuses scanned before 20 weeks' gestation (Whittle 1997). The decision to investigate the karyotype of affected fetuses is not clear cut. Some authors (Donnenfeld 1995) conclude that because such cysts are associated with the aneuploidy trisomy 18, infants with which rarely survive past 5 months, it is not worth the risk or cost of amniocentesis. Conversely, Walkinshaw *et al.* (1994) conclude that the presence of choroid plexus cysts in fetuses beyond 19 weeks' gestation should be investigated through karyotyping as their study showed that, where choroid plexus cysts were the only marker, trisomy was diagnosed in 1 out of 82 cases. This conclusion is also supported by the later work of Chew *et al.* (1995).

According to information derived from a meta-analysis of over 1400 reported cases of choroid plexus cysts worldwide (Gupta *et al.* 1995), the risk of chromosomal abnormality increases to approximately 1 in 3 when combined with the detection of other ultrasound anomalies. Risk is not related to the size of the cysts or whether they are unilateral or bilateral.

NUCHAL TRANSLUCENCY

In a multicentre study at the Harris Birthright Centre and four district general hospitals 20,804 pregnancies were included in nuchal screening at 10–14 weeks' gestation (Snijders *et al.* 1996). It was demonstrated that 80% of affected fetuses with trisomy 21 could be identified through using this method with a false-positive rate of 5%.

PYELECTASIS

Dilated renal pelves are detectable using ultrasound and may be indicative of an abnormal urinary tract. In a study by Adra *et al.* (1995), renal pathology was confirmed at birth in 44% of pyelectasis cases identified antenatally, the most common features being ureteropelvic junction obstruction and vesicoureteral reflux. All cases of pyelectasis should be referred to a urologist for evaluation after birth.

The triple/double/Bart's test

In 1988 a test was developed by researchers at St Bartholomew's Hospital which was based on maternal serum, and hence carried no risk to the developing fetus. It became available in 1989, and, known as the triple test, is now widely available in maternity units. This test is

TABLE 3.1 Maternal serum markers in the triple test

Alphafetoprotein (AFP)	Reduced levels
Oestriol (E$_3$)	Reduced levels
Human chorionic gonadotrophin (hCG)	Increased levels

usually carried out between 14 and 16 weeks' gestation and is based on the combined picture provided by three markers (Table 3.1).

The results are adjusted according to gestational age and maternal weight. Other factors that are known to affect the interpretation of the results include maternal smoking, ethnic origin and diabetes. Unlike amniocentesis, the test does not provide prospective parents with a definite result, but a calculated 'risk' for that individual pregnancy.

The test is usually offered on the basis that the woman accepts that further investigations are normally only offered if her result falls into a high-risk category and this is predetermined at a certain ratio. For example, her individual risk of having a baby with Down's syndrome may come back as 1 in 250. The hospital may have a policy to offer further tests to women who have a risk of 1 in 200 or more. Thus she spends the rest of her pregnancy knowing that she has a relatively high risk of giving birth to a Down's syndrome child, and her decision to have the screening test has not provided any reassurance but instead created doubt and uncertainty.

Of course, the above situation is only one example of how screening for abnormality can raise more questions than it answers. However, the triple test can provide useful information to women who would previously have fallen into the category for routine amniocentesis because of their age. Such women may have a triple test which yields a very low risk for her as an individual, rather than the blanket risk which could have been cited based on age alone, and she therefore opts not to have an amniocentesis, avoiding the potential risk of miscarriage this test carries.

Amniocentesis

Amniocentesis involves the collection of a sample of amniotic fluid, from which fetal cells are cultured and abnormalities identified. Performed under ultrasound guidance, a pocket of fluid is identified and approximately 10–20 ml of fluid is withdrawn. It carries with it the risk of miscarriage in about 1 in 200 pregnancies, although this will vary between individual operators. This risk is calculated against the fact that a definite result can be given whether or not a baby is affected by a particular condition, and management can be based on this knowledge.

Unfortunately, because this test relies upon a significant amount of liquor being present, it cannot normally be performed before about 16 weeks' gestation. It also requires the culturing of fetal cells which takes about 3 weeks. Therefore, should a termination of pregnancy be indicated, it would be taking place at almost 20 weeks of pregnancy, by which time fetal movements have usually been felt, the baby has been seen on the ultrasound screen and the pregnancy is noticeable to outside eyes.

Rothman (1988) describes how the situation of getting to know the developing baby through the amniocentesis procedure makes the decision to terminate the pregnancy after an abnormal result so difficult for women.

Women who have had a termination for abnormality in a previous pregnancy may relive their feelings of guilt and sorrow after the birth of their subsequent offspring, and the practitioner needs to be sensitive to this and respectful of that decision.

Subsequent antenatal care

The schedule of antenatal care has changed in recent years to reflect the individual needs of women. The pattern of care in the United Kingdom was originally set out in the 1929 report from the Ministry of Health and stated that visits should be fortnightly from 28 weeks and weekly from 36 weeks of pregnancy. What, in the past, was very regimented and concrete is now much more flexible and client centred. This change was initiated by work undertaken by Hall (1980), which highlighted the fact that many women with uncomplicated pregnancies were being seen routinely. Change is still in its infancy, however, and many women remember how often they were seen in previous pregnancies and are reluctant to give up their antenatal checks. In an intervention study conducted by Sikorski *et al.* (1996), 2,794 women were randomly allocated to either traditional care (13 visits) or 'new style' (seven visits). The outcomes evaluated included satisfaction and clinical variables. The results showed that in reality the difference between the two groups in terms of the number of visits they actually received was less than anticipated (10.8 compared with 8.6). Although there was no statistical significance between the clinical variables, women were more dissatisfied if they were in the study group, women valuing regular contact with professionals.

While this debate goes on, the content of antenatal care has changed very little and comprises the following routine assessment:

- fundal height
- fetal heart rate
- fetal movements
- fetal position
- urinalysis
- assessment for oedema
- blood pressure measurement.

It is policy in some maternity units to undertake a formal risk assessment for all pregnant women. However, this procedure has a low sensitivity in terms of identifying pregnancies that subsequently develop problems, and only a small proportion of pregnancies that are categorised as high risk will actually result in complications.

The purpose of each component of the antenatal examination will now be summarised, enabling the practitioner to appreciate the relevance of such measurements to the examination of the newborn infant.

Fundal height is used to assess fetal growth. It is often performed by an experienced practitioner using anatomical landmarks. However, it is also suggested that the distance from the symphysis to the fundus, when measured in centimetres using a tape measure, is a useful (although imprecise) diagnostic tool for the detection of light for gestational age infants (Stuart *et al*. 1989). Deviation from the expected height for gestation should be investigated further by means of an ultrasound scan.

If a fetus is suspected of either being light or large for gestational age, a series of scans is conducted in order to assess fetal growth over time. Measurements are made of head circumference and abdominal girth, from which an estimate of fetal weight can be made.

It is important therefore that the practitioner is alert to the recorded antenatal growth pattern in order to make an accurate diagnosis of the babies health status at birth. For clinical factors associated with large for gestational age and small for gestational age babies compared with the preterm infant see Chapters 5 and 6.

Fetal heart rate is first identified using ultrasound at approximately 6 weeks of amenorrhoea; thereafter it is detectable via electronic means as soon as the fundus is palpable abdominally. The normal fetal heart rate is between 120 and 160 beats per minute, although this will vary during rest, activity, maternal drug therapy, maternal tachycardia and venacaval compression.

Occasionally, an abnormal rhythm is detected antenatally and if confirmed would require specialist referral before delivery. The fetal heart rate is also recorded when a cardiotocography (CTG) is performed.

Fetal movements are a simple measure showing that the fetus has an adequate oxygen supply in order to exercise its muscles. When reduced fetal movements are reported they are investigated by cardiotocography (CTG), which examines not only the fetal heart rate but also the ability of the fetus to respond to an increased demand for oxygen.

Fetal position is recorded in the last weeks of pregnancy. If the baby has been in a particular position antenatally, it may have sequelae for the examination of the newborn. For example, if the baby has been in a posterior position the baby's head may be temporarily elongated, which may be alarming for the parents. A baby who was presenting by the breech may continue to extend its leg for a few days. Although this is perfectly normal, it will test the nappy changing skills of new parents!

Urinalysis is undertaken at each antenatal visit and may detect glycosuria (this may occur in a macrosomic infant) or proteinuria (may indicate hypertension or infection)

Blood pressure is also measured at each antenatal visit. If the blood pressure is raised in addition to proteinuria (with or without oedema), the woman is said to have pregnancy-induced hypertension. Subsequently, her baby may be small for gestational age and labour may also have been induced before full term. The practitioner examining the baby may therefore need to be prepared to discuss the relevance of this condition to the baby and provide general reassurance.

We have considered the routine content of antenatal care; however, occasionally additional tests have been applied during the antenatal period.

Additional tests

Biophysical profile

This test for assessment of fetal wellbeing involves ultrasound scanning by a skilled operator. In a similar way to the Apgar score, it combines examination of a number of parameters and a score out of 2 for each of the following is given.

Fetal heart rate	Fetal breathing movements
Pockets of liquor	Fetal tone
Placental grading (optional)	Doppler (optional)

A score of less than 7 is associated with decreased fetal wellbeing (Sherer *et al.* 1996) and can play a valuable part in the decision to expedite delivery. In a retrospective study, Manning *et al.* (1998) concluded that antenatal biophysical profiling is associated with a significant reduction in the incidence of cerebral palsy compared with untested patients.

Cordocentesis

This procedure involves the removal of fetal blood via the umbilical cord during pregnancy. It is rarely undertaken but may provide vital information in cases such as rhesus isoimmunisation. Transfusions can also be given *in utero*. It would be the remit of a senior paediatrician to examine any neonate who had been 'at risk' antenatally.

Summary

It has been shown that there are a range of antenatal parameters that the practitioner examining the neonate should be aware of in order to be sensitive to the needs of the mother and her baby. Detailed examination of the booking history details and subsequent antenatal records are an essential component of the examination of the newborn. The next chapter considers the impact of events during labour and childbirth on the health of the neonate.

Chapter 4

Risks to the fetus during childbirth

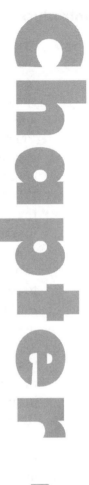

Introduction

We have already considered the various risks that the developing fetus may encounter during the antenatal period and how these have relevance for the examination of the newborn baby (Chapter 3). However, it should be acknowledged that the perfectly healthy term baby may be affected by how the labour and delivery progressed and were managed. Practitioners should therefore possess a thorough knowledge of labour and delivery, the difficulties that can arise in childbirth and their possible consequences for the health of the newborn. The events surrounding the birth will be carefully documented in the mother's records, and these should be scrutinised in advance so that the examination takes into account any increased risk factors associated with a particular birth. It is important that practitioners are fully aware of the events surrounding each labour and delivery in order to respond appropriately to parents who may, for a number of reasons, have concerns relating to the birth of their child. Although it is acknowledged that midwives and neonatal nurses often care for neonates requiring additional care, such as premature infants or those with feeding difficulties, it should be noted that only healthy, full-term neonates should be clinically examined by the midwife. All other cases should be referred to a medical practitioner, in line with local policy (see Chapter 7) and professional guidance (UKCC 1998).

Having ensured that this particular examination of the newborn falls within the practitioner's remit, the following questions should be borne in mind:

1 Was the pregnancy prolonged?
2 Was the labour induced or accelerated, and if so why?
3 How long were the fetal membranes ruptured prior to delivery?
4 Were there any anomalies of the fetal heart rate during labour?
5 Was the liquor meconium stained?
6 What were the methods of pain relief used during the labour and birth?
7 What was the presenting part of the fetus during labour?
8 What was the mode of delivery?
9 Did the baby require any resuscitation at birth?
10 Were any injuries or abnormalities noted at the birth?

This chapter will focus on outlining the relevance of these questions to the health of the baby, enabling the practitioner to conduct a thorough and effective examination.

Prolonged pregnancy

The practitioner examining the newborn baby needs to have an awareness of the current perspectives regarding prolonged pregnancy so that women who question the management of their labour understand the rationale behind it. Such knowledge also helps the practitioner put into context some of the problems that they might encounter in the neonate.

Prolonged or post-term pregnancy is defined by the International Federation of Gynaecology and Obstetrics (FIGO 1984) as more than 42 completed weeks of pregnancy and has long been associated with poor perinatal outcome. A study conducted by Divon *et al.* (1998) detected a significant rise in the odds ratio for fetal mortality from 41 or more weeks' gestation, but no significant rise for neonatal mortality. Hilder *et al.* (1998) in their analysis of 171,527 notified births found an increase in stillbirth and infant mortality from 0.7 per 1000 ongoing pregnancies at 37 weeks to 5.8 per 1000 ongoing pregnancies at 43 weeks' gestation, signifying an eightfold increase. The aetiology of prolonged pregnancy is complex and is thought to include factors such as congenital abnormalities that interfere with the fetal pituitary–adrenal axis and environmental contributors such as diet and pollution (Shea *et al.* 1998).

In terms of morbidity, the outlook for the baby of prolonged gestation is generally good because of many factors, including accurate estimation of gestational age using ultrasonography, early intervention after heart rate anomalies in labour and close monitoring of post-term pregnancies (Campbell 1998). However, in a study conducted by Roach and Rogers (1997) it was found that, although there was no increase in mortality before 42 weeks' gestation in pregnancies being monitored (through serial monitoring of amniotic fluid index and cardiotocography), after 42 weeks there was an increased Caesarean section rate and incidence of meconium identified below the vocal cords. The incidence of meconium-stained liquor increases with postmaturity and may be considered to be an indication for inducing labour post term in order to avoid meconium aspiration (Adhikari *et al.* 1998).

The management of post-term pregnancy is a careful balance between the risks of postmaturity and the risks associated with induction of labour. A review of the literature published in *Drugs and Therapeutic Bulletin* (1997) concluded that routine induction of labour at 42 weeks' gestation is associated with a lower risk of perinatal death. A study by Sarker and Hill (1996) associates prolonged pregnancy with a significantly higher level of maternal anxiety antenatally, and this may have an impact on maternal wellbeing in the postnatal period that the examiner should be aware of.

The post-term infant is generally a baby that feeds well and requires little special attention in the postnatal period. They have characteristically dry skin that may be prone to cracking, and parents can be advised to massage the baby with a neutral vegetable oil, which the baby will enjoy, and to avoid using soap-based products when bathing the baby. It may have long fingernails and is therefore likely to scratch itself, although extreme caution should be used if attempting to trim them because the nail is usually joined to the very tip of the finger in young babies. The use of special scissors under the control of a clear-sighted adult is recommended.

Induction of labour

The importance of the practitioner exploring this issue with regard to the neonatal examination is twofold;

1 The *rationale* for the induction can be followed through, for example, if labour was induced because the mother had pregnancy-induced hypertension, and what has been the effect on the baby.
2 The effect on the fetus of the *method* of induction used can be anticipated.

Labour is induced for a variety of reasons, including postmaturity, large or small for gestational age fetus, diabetes, pregnancy-induced hypertension, prolonged rupture of membranes and individual social circumstances. Babies with specific problems will be managed under the care of a paediatrician.

Induction of labour often involves the administration of oxytocin via an intravenous infusion. There has been some debate regarding a link between its use and the incidence of neonatal jaundice (Chen 1992, Woyton *et al.* 1994), although, according to Johnson *et al.* (1984), this effect may be more to do with the large volume of sodium solution received by the mother during its administration. Whatever the aetiology, it would be worth preparing the mother for the possibility of the baby becoming jaundiced in terms of what look out for in her baby's appearance and its behaviour (see Chapter 6).

The risk of precipitate delivery is also increased after induced labour, especially in multigravid women. The practitioner examining the baby must therefore be diligent to exclude the possibility of a tentorial tear caused by rapid moulding of the fetal skull, although such babies would usually be born in a state of shock.

Prolonged and premature rupture of the membranes

Premature rupture of the membranes (PROMs) is defined as rupture of the fetal membranes before the onset of labour and occurs in about 10% of all pregnancies; 90% of these are at term (Alexander and Cox 1996). PROMs at term is managed by either induction of labour or expectant management if there are no signs of maternal or neonatal morbidity. Prolonged rupture of the fetal membranes (> 24 hours) has long been associated with maternal and neonatal infection, and this issue has been the subject of debate for many years (Beckwith and Read 1996).

A study conducted by Ottervanger et al. (1996), which compared expectant management (48 hours) of prelabour rupture of the membranes with induction of labour, found that those women randomised to induction were more likely to have an operative delivery and require analgesia in labour, but that there was no difference between the rate of neonatal or maternal infection. These results concur with those of Hannah et al. (1996), whose randomised controlled trial involving 5,041 women found that the overall rate of neonatal infection where the membranes ruptured before labour was 2.6%. There was no difference in the incidence of neonatal infection rates between the four study groups, but maternal satisfaction was lower in the expectant management groups.

The number of vaginal examinations that the woman is likely to have performed on her following prelabour rupture of the membranes may be linked to infection rates. In one study (Ladfors et al. 1996) comparing two methods of expectant management of prelabour rupture of the membranes, a protocol of infrequent vaginal examinations was associated with low maternal and fetal infection. This result was echoed in the study by Hannah et al. (1996), which linked fewer vaginal examinations with a low rate of maternal infection.

We have seen from the literature that premature rupture of the membranes at term, in the absence of signs and symptoms of infection, does not present a serious risk to the neonate. This does not mean, however, that the practitioner examining the newborn can be complacent about premature rupture of the membranes, especially when working within a unit that actively manages such cases. Despite the evidence, it is the practice in many maternity units to induce labour if it does not establish within 24 hours of membrane rupture. Some units also take swabs from the neonate in order to exclude infection if delivery is more than 24 hours after rupture of the membranes, but particularly if maternal infection is verified or the liquor was foul smelling. If swabs have been taken, there must be a system for the follow-up of positive results, and the practitioner should endeavour to establish the baby's status and make a record of it. While swab results are awaited, it would be prudent to explain to parents how to recognise the signs and symptoms of infection (Chapter 6) and to inform the relevant personnel in the domiciliary setting of all action taken.

Anomalies of the fetal heart rate in labour

Continuous fetal heart rate monitoring during labour was introduced in the 1970s, before it had been shown to lead to improvements in neonatal outcome. In fact, there is evidence from subsequent randomised controlled trials (Kelso *et al*. 1978, Haverkamp *et al*. 1979, MacDonald *et al*. 1985) that electronic fetal monitoring (EFM) increases the risk of Caesarean section and operative vaginal delivery. EFM has been shown to reduce the risk of neonatal seizures, but at further follow-up these babies did not suffer any long-term damage as a result (MacDonald *et al*. 1985). Despite the availability of systematic reviews of the relevant trials (Enkin *et al*. 1995), EFM remains part of the labour ritual in many delivery suites.

EFM does detect abnormal fetal heart rate patterns but its specificity is poor. It can show bradycardia, tachycardia, reduced variability and reduced response to stimuli. Many fit and healthy babies, however, have been delivered by emergency Caesarean section on the basis of an 'abnormal' fetal heart rate pattern. Unnecessary intervention is less likely to occur if EFM is used in conjunction with fetal blood sampling (FBS) in order to establish the pH of the fetal blood (Table 4.1) (Lissauer and Steer 1986).

Pulse oximetry is being investigated as a less invasive alternative to FBS (Carbonne 1997). The parents of a baby whose delivery was expedited on the basis of such findings may require reassurance from the professional undertaking the first examination of the newborn that their baby has not suffered any long-term damage due to lack of oxygen

TABLE 4.1 pH of fetal scalp blood

Investigation	Normal	Borderline	Abnormal
Fetal scalp blood pH	7.25	7.20–7.24	7.19 or less

during the birth. It would be a valuable exercise to take them step by step through the examination, highlighting what you are looking for. It is not possible at this stage to say *categorically* that the baby is perfect, but that you have not identified any cause for concern.

A point to note is that use of internal fetal scalp electrodes, to record fetal heart rate patterns, has been associated with trauma to the baby's scalp (Akhter 1976), and the practitioner examining the baby should ensure that they observe any puncture site and carefully document the findings.

Meconium-stained liquor

We have already seen that the incidence of meconium-stained liquor increases with maturity. The mature infant is also more likely to make attempts to breathe when depleted of oxygen and therefore is more likely to inhale substances present in the birth canal, such as vernix, blood and meconium. This situation – the hypoxic mature infant surrounded by meconium-stained liquor – increases the possibility that the baby will aspirate meconium. Meconium aspiration may lead to meconium aspiration syndrome (MAS), a potentially fatal condition during which the baby has severe respiratory difficulties and requires admission to a neonatal unit.

Babies who have been exposed to meconium-stained liquor but who are not suspected of having inhaled meconium are observed on the postnatal ward. The respiration rate is recorded hourly for the first 4–6 hours and abnormalities must be reported to a paediatrician. The practitioner should also observe the baby for signs of infection as this has been associated with meconium-stained liquor, especially thick meconium (Piper *et al.* 1998).

Pharmacological pain relief

The impact on the neonate of the type of pain relief used by the mother in labour will be influenced by the following factors:

- type of drug(s) used
- dose(s) given
- route of administration of the drug
- stage of labour drug administered
- weight of the baby
- maturity of the baby.

The therapeutic range of a drug is calculated using the body mass index. The smaller the baby the greater the effect of the drug.

The practitioner examining the baby will need to consider all of the above when reading the woman's labour and delivery records in order to assess how this history may affect the neonate. The effects on the baby of the drugs commonly used in labour will be outlined in the following sections.

Entonox

Entonox (50% nitrous oxide/50% oxygen) is inhaled by the mother. This drug is excreted by the mother's lungs and therefore the amount that enters her bloodstream, and hence crosses the placenta, is negligible.

Narcotic drugs

Pethidine is commonly administered to the mother for pain relief in the first stage of labour, although its effectiveness has been questioned (Olofsson *et al*. 1996). This drug is given by intramuscular injection to the mother, is absorbed into her bloodstream and crosses the placenta. Dosage ranges from 50 to 150 mg and is usually given every 3–4 hours. Pethidine has a half-life of 5 hours in the mother and it is metabolised in the liver; but as the neonatal liver is immature, the effects on the neonate are prolonged (Gamsu 1993). It is a narcotic and therefore depresses respiratory effort. Respiratory depression in the baby can be effectively reversed at delivery by administering naloxone intramuscularly in addition to establishing airway patency and oxygenation.

The more insidious effects on the baby of lethargy and the lack of interest to feed are also of concern, especially in the breast feeding baby. Breast feeding can be an emotional issue, and a mother who is experiencing difficulties with a baby who does not appear interested in feeding will need support. The practitioner examining the baby can encourage the mother in the above situation that the baby's response is likely to be a consequence of the pethidine she received in labour, and that it is therefore worth persevering. It must be acknowledged, however, that in the first 24 hours after delivery the baby will in fact get an extra dose of pethidine via the mother's breast milk, but that thereafter this effect will decline (Freeborn *et al.* 1980). Morphine is also a narcotic drug used in labour, but less frequently than pethidine.

Epidural

In a study conducted by Lieberman *et al.* (1997) involving 1,657 women it was concluded that neonates whose mothers received epidurals in labour were more likely to require treatment with antibiotics. This may be related to the fact that epidural analgesia in labour has been associated with an increase in maternal temperature (Mercier and Benhamou 1997), which may lead to the precautionary measure of admitting her baby to a special care baby unit with suspected infection (Pleasure and Stahl 1990). In general, however, epidural use in labour is not associated with a poor neonatal outcome and is the preferred method of anaesthesia for Caesarean section.

Water birth

In many maternity units a birthing pool is available for women to use for its analgesic effects. There is no evidence to suggest that such an option for women results in a higher risk to the neonate (Alderice *et al.* 1995, Brown 1998). An unusual case of neonatal polycythaemia was reported (Odent 1998) in an infant who remained in a birthing pool for 30 minutes after delivery before the cord was cut; when a baby is born on dry land, the effect of the air causes the cord to constrict thereby limiting the amount of blood transfused from the placenta.

Presentation of the fetus in labour

Knowledge of how the fetus presented during labour and its relevance to the clinical examination is required so that the practitioner can reassure parents and look for specific features. The following presentations will be considered:

1 occipito-posterior
2 face
3 brow
4 compound
5 breech.

Occipito-posterior

This is a relatively common presentation, affecting approximately 10% of babies (Bennett and Brown 1999). Moulding of the fetal skull results in a characteristically elongated head, which resolves in a few days.

Face presentation

For vaginal delivery to take place this requires the fetus to extend its head and neck. The face is usually very bruised and may have a circular demarcation on it (caused by the pressure of the cervix) if there was any delay in labour.

Brow presentation

This rarely delivers vaginally unless the baby is small and the pelvis large. The characteristic moulding results in an elongated sinciput and occiput, with the top of the head appearing flattened.

Compound presentation

This occurs when a hand or foot lies along side the head. During the delivery the operator may have manipulated the limb over the baby's face resulting in bruising or swelling.

Breech

The breech presents in approximately 3% of all term pregnancies. Many are delivered by elective Caesarean section, and this is a matter of on-going debate. A retrospective study conducted in Sweden (Lindqvist *et al.* 1997) supports the view that there is no increased perinatal mortality in term vaginal breech deliveries compared with those delivered by Caesarean section. The inadequate training of doctors at registrar level to conduct vaginal breech deliveries has been associated with an increase in the number of Caesarean sections performed for breech presentation (Sharma *et al.* 1997).

Breech babies, if born vaginally, may have bruised and swollen genitals, the appearance of which are distressing for parents. If the baby was an extended breech, it will lie in the cot with its legs extended for a few days. Parents should be encouraged to clean and handle the baby as usual (although changing the nappy is quite difficult!) and the baby's unusual position will gradually resolve.

Congenital dislocation of the hips is also a potential complication of babies that have presented by the breech position. In an Australian study of 1,127 cases of congenital dislocated hips, the risk associated with breech presentation was estimated to be 2.7% for girls and 0.8% for boys (Chan *et al.* 1997).

The head of the breech baby is characteristically round as there has been a rapid journey through the birth canal with little time for moulding. The shape of the baby's head is a positive outcome of undergoing an unusual delivery, which the practitioner might like to comment on during the examination for the benefit of the parents.

Mode of delivery

This section will outline the normal neonatal outcomes after instrumental and operative deliveries. It is important to note that a paediatrician is not always present at instrumental and operative deliveries, depending on the indication and type of anaesthesia used. The first examination of the newborn may, therefore, be the first time that the baby is clinically examined, unless there were any indications. One study (Jacob and Pfenninger 1997) found that the use of regional anaesthesia for elective or non-urgent Caesarean sections reduced the incidence of vigorous resuscitation (defined as bag and mask ventilation, tracheal intubation and cardiopulmonary resuscitation) to a level similar to that of vaginal delivery.

Instrumental delivery is the course of action that follows a complication of pregnancy during labour. The examiner will therefore need to consider the relevance of that complication to the baby's health. If the delivery was expedited for prolonged labour, for example, is there an indication for screening the baby for infection? When surveying the mother's notes, the practitioner will need to consider the following points:

- indication for intervention;
- how long had the mother been in labour prior to intervention; and
- what was the condition of the baby at delivery.

Unfortunately, not all women have the opportunity to talk through the events of their labour and delivery with the midwife or doctor who was there. This is especially important when events do not go according to plan. In most cases women will have been sufficiently informed and involved in their care to have a clear understanding of what actually happened and why. There will be some women who, either because of the stress of the moment or through the haze of sedation, do not know exactly what happened at the birth. She may turn to the practitioner examining her baby for an explanation of events. Unless it is *absolutely* clear from the delivery records why, for example, she needed an emergency forceps delivery, always refer her to either the midwife who was at the delivery or her obstetrician. Do not attempt to answer questions that you do not know the answers to, but do ensure that she does have the opportunity to see someone who can answer them.

Some maternity units offer a debriefing service for women after childbirth (Smith and Mitchell 1996), but this is variable. The term 'post traumatic stress disorder' is increasingly being applied to women's distress after an event in childbirth (Crompton 1996), and it must be acknowledged that women may need information and support in order to come to terms with events (Allott 1996).

Ventouse and forceps delivery

Ventouse delivery is the preferred method when assisted vaginal delivery is required (Chalmers and Chalmers 1989). The neonate may suffer damage to the scalp after a ventouse delivery. The anticipated swelling is referred to as a chignon and may be accompanied by bruising and abrasion. Such trauma will be dependent on whether a soft or a metal cup was used, how many times the cup was reapplied, how many pulls were used, and these factors will themselves be dependent on the protocol of the unit and the skill of the operator. A systematic review of the evidence comparing forceps with ventouse (Johanson and Menon 2000) concluded that, in relation to the baby:

- the vacuum extractor is associated with more cephalhaematomata (see Chapter 6);

- women worry more about the condition of their baby with the ventouse;
- forceps leads to more facial and cranial injuries;
- there is no difference in number of babies requiring phototherapy; and
- there is no difference in re-admission rates between the two instruments.

Caesarean section

The Caesarean section rate varies between consultants, units and countries and is divided between those that are conducted in an emergency and those that are elective.

A complication for the baby after abdominal delivery is laceration during surgery. According to a retrospective review of the neonatal records of 904 Caesarean deliveries (Smith *et al.* 1997), the incidence of lacerations was 1.9% ($n = 17$). The incidence was higher in non-vertex presentation (6% compared with 1.4% of vertex) and only one of the 17 lacerations was documented in the maternal notes, possibly indicating that obstetricians were unaware of this complication.

The practitioner examining the baby may discover a laceration during the examination which had previously gone unnoticed. It is important not to attempt to hide such a discovery from the parents, but to explain that this is a complication of Caesarean section due to the close proximity of the fetus to the uterine wall. The significance of a laceration to the parents should not be undermined, especially if it is on the babies face, but most parents can balance this with the relief that their baby's delivery was expedited to avoid a much more serious outcome. The obstetrician who conducted the delivery should be informed of the laceration and careful records made. Such wounds are usually clean and heal quickly with the aid of a steri-strip. A red scar may persist for some weeks but will eventually fade and become unnoticeable.

Babies born by Caesarean section have an increased risk of developing transient tachypnoea of the newborn (TTN) caused by delayed absorption of alveolar fluid. This condition may require oxygen therapy (Seidel *et al.* 1997) and admission to a special care baby unit.

Resuscitation at birth

During your scrutiny of the mother's delivery details, it is important to note the condition of the baby at delivery in order that you may anticipate potential questions from the parents. All babies are given an Apgar score at delivery, but this is not always conveyed to the parents. It is not appropriate that in your role as examiner of the healthy newborn infant that you will be called upon to examine the severely birth-asphyxiated baby; such a baby would be carefully monitored in a neonatal unit. You will, however, examine babies who did require some form of resuscitation at birth, including administration of oxygen, oropharyngeal suction and intramuscular injection.

Resuscitation procedures are undertaken regularly by nurses, midwives and paediatricians. They are not, however, part of the daily repertoire of parents and can be alarming and confusing. The practitioner examining the baby can very simply clarify the confusion by saying, for example, 'I see from your notes that Hannah needed some oxygen when she was born because she did not want to breathe at first. She had some oxygen through a facemask and she became lovely and pink straight away. Her Apgar scores were fine (explaining what they are) and she came back to you. Is there anything you want to ask?' Such an explanation also reassures the parents that you know details about their daughter and are taking a thorough approach to her examination.

Injuries and abnormalities noticed at birth

It has already been seen that during the course of their delivery some babies sustain an injury, such as a chignon, and these are discussed in more detail in Chapter 6. The purpose of mentioning them in the context of the first examination of the newborn is to remind the examiner to evaluate how the condition is progressing and that it is remaining within the limits of normality. Recognising that abnormality has been detected at birth, such as a birth mark, enables the practitioner to allocate a realistic length of time for the examination so that parents can ask extra questions that may have come to mind overnight. Parents may also need further information regarding subsequent care, and where possible this should be reinforced through the availability of high-quality written information. National support groups for parents with children who have congenital abnormalities are detailed in Appendix 1.

Summary

Careful exploration of the delivery records provides a wealth of valuable detail that will help with the examination of the newborn. It enables the examiner to provide personal, client-focused care and enhances the effectiveness of the procedure. As with all aspects of clinical practice, the practitioner must acknowledge when they are out of their depth and not attempt to deal with questions that they are not able to answer comprehensively.

The next chapter provides the reader with a systematic guide to undertaking the clinical examination of the healthy, term neonate and is the foundation from which normality can be confirmed and abnormality detected.

Chapter 5

Neonatal examination

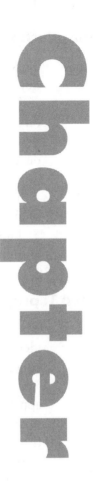

- Introduction
- Step 1: preparation
- Step 2: observation
- Step 3: examination
- Step 4: explanation to the parent(s)
- Step 5: documentation

Introduction

This chapter is a step-by-step guide to the first examination of the newborn. It will take the practitioner systematically through the process and introduce the principles of the neonatal examination. It will focus on the normal expected findings and also describe the abnormal findings that *may* be detected. It is through anticipation of the normal that deviations are detected, and this is the philosophy of the examination described in this chapter.

It is not within the remit of this chapter to discuss the management of abnormalities – this will be addressed in Chapter 6.

This chapter will describe five steps: preparation, observation, examination, explanation and documentation (Table 5.1).

Step 1: preparation

The antenatal and labour records should be carefully scrutinised to identify any factors that might lead the practitioner to suspect potential concerns, as detailed in Chapters 2, 3 and 4 (for summary, see Table 5.2). This preparation is also important so that the practitioner can approach the parents with an accurate history of what has happened to them, demonstrating that time and care have been taken to focus on this unique family unit.

Before the neonate is disturbed, a great deal can be learned by listening to those who are caring for the mother and the baby (Table 5.3). It is also important to gather together the equipment that will be required during the examination and to ensure that it is clean and in working order. The following is a list of equipment required to perform the neonatal examination:

- stethoscope
- ophthalmoscope
- spatula
- tape measure
- stadiometer (or equivalent)
- centile chart.

To have to leave the bedside to search for equipment might result in a previously contented baby becoming unsettled, hungry or in need of comfort, and the examination would then need to be postponed.

TABLE 5.1 The five steps of neonatal examination

Step	Action	Description
1	Preparation	Read case notes (Table 5.2) Listen to carers (Table 5.3) Gather equipment Wash and warm hands
2	Observation	Watch baby's behaviour Listen to the baby Listen to the mother
3	Examination	Baby dressed Baby undressed
4	Explanation	Findings conveyed to mother
5	Documentation	Examination and action documented

Whoever performs the examination must be familiar with the art of clinical examination, which should always include the same four components:

- looking (inspection)
- feeling (palpation)
- listening (auscultation)
- tapping (percussion).

The first and third components are self-explanatory, but the second and fourth require explanation of how they are performed, depending on which part of the baby is being examined. Immediately before examining the baby the practitioner's hands should be washed and warmed.

Palpation is best performed with warm hands. It can give information about the firmness of underlying tissue, e.g. bony or cystic, the transmission of sound, e.g. murmurs or breath sounds, the size of and position of organs and the presence of masses. Palpation is performed differently depending on the situation; therefore, specific instructions will be given at the relevant points in the chapter.

Percussion can usually differentiate solid or fluid-filled tissue from gas-filled tissue. It is performed by placing the middle finger of the left hand flat on the baby's body and gently tapping the middle phalanx with the middle finger of the right hand. This technique can be useful

TABLE 5.2 Points to look for in the notes

Problem/disorder type	Example(s)
Family history	
Cardiac	Hypertrophic obstructive cardiomyopathy
Chromosome-related syndromes	Balanced translocation(s)
Developmental	Congenital deafness
Endocrine	Congenital adrenal hypo- or hyperplasia
Haematological	Haemoglobinopathies
Locomotor	Congenital dislocation of the hip
Metabolic	Galactosaemia
Neurodegenerative	Baton's disease
Neuromuscular	Spinomuscular dystrophy
Respiratory	Cystic fibrosis
Tumours	Retinoblastoma
Past medical history	
Endocrine	Graves' disease, congenital hypothyroidism and diabetes
Haematological	Isoimmune thrombocytopenic purpura
Hypertension	Essential/pregnancy induced
Neuromuscular	Myasthenia gravis
Psychiatric	Postnatal depression
Medication	Teratogens, e.g. anticonvulsants, stilboestrol, thalidomide
Past obstetric history	
Anomalies/disorders	Pre-term labour
Deaths	Sudden infant death
Infection	Cytomegalovirus
Social	Adoption/fostering
Present obstetric history	
Expected date of delivery	Is the baby full term?
Conception	Donor
Habits	Alcohol, nicotine and drugs
Infection	Group B *Streptococcus*, hepatitis B and C, herpes
Size	Abnormal/asymmetrical growth
Monitoring	Anomaly scans, glycosuria

Delivery details

Cardiotocograph anomalies	Decelerations
Delivery type and reason	Emergency section for fetal distress
Duration of membrane rupture	Prolonged rupture
Maternal medication	Opiates
Maternal wellbeing	Pyrexia

Baby

Condition of baby at birth	Apnoeic
Evidence of distress	Meconium passage *in utero*
Resuscitation details	Apgar scores, ventilatory support
Feeding	Breast/bottle
Vitamin K administered	Oral/intramuscular

TABLE 5.3 Points to listen for from carers

	Observation(s)	*Example(s)*
Baby	Behaviour	Jittery, irritable, sleepy, etc.
	Feeding	Vomiting
	Monitoring	Pyrexia, colour, etc.
Mother	Behaviour generally	Tearful
	Behaviour towards baby	Caring, rough

for examination of the chest (the percussion note is hyper-resonant in the presence of a pneumothorax) and abdomen.

Step 2: observation

In addition, much can be learned about the neonate by looking and listening to him before disturbing him (Table 5.4). It is also wise to listen to the mother, who will already be the best judge of her baby's behaviour. Once all the information has been gathered from these sources, the neonate can be disturbed.

Step 3: examination

Examination of the baby is best performed with the (right-handed) practitioner standing on the right-hand side of the bed with the baby lying with its head to the left of the practitioner.

One of the most difficult and important systems to examine is the

Table 5.4 Observations before disturbing the neonate

Observation(s)	Example(s) of abnormalities
Colour	Cyanosis, pallor, plethora, jaundice
Cry	High pitched
Movement	Jittery, asymmetry
Posture	Hypotonia, Erb's palsy
Respiration	Recession, grunting, apnoea

heart, for the baby must be calm and content. It is therefore prudent to examine the heart first. Initially, the neonate should be observed for cyanosis. His respiratory pattern should also be observed. The next steps are palpation and auscultation. Traditionally, these steps are performed with the neonate undressed, but beware, for although the neonate is born naked, he soon finds security in the closeness of clothing and removal of that clothing can result in a crying neonate. Under these circumstances, palpation and auscultation may not reveal any useful information about the heart. In the first instance, it is worth attempting to palpate the chest and auscultate the heart with the neonate partially clothed. Successful auscultation of the heart sounds with the baby partially clothed does not preclude further examination of him when he is naked. However, if he then cries inconsolably when you undress him, at least the heart sounds will have been heard and the presence of louder murmurs excluded.

Before undressing the neonate, it also pays to concentrate next on the exposed parts of the baby (Table 5.5) and those areas which would be best examined before the practitioner puts her hands into a nappy full of meconium, i.e. eyes and mouth.

Once the exposed parts of the baby have been examined thoroughly the neonate may be undressed and the final stage of the examination begun (Table 5.6).

Scalp

The scalp is most commonly the presenting part at delivery. It is relatively easily traumatised and swelling with or without bruising is relatively common. A cranial meningocele or encephalocele may also produce a swelling. The scalp is also a common site for birthmarks or other skin abnormalities.

TABLE 5.5 Exposed parts of the baby

Part of body	Abnormalities to look out for
Scalp	Bruising/swelling
Head	Sutures and fontanelles Size Asymmetry/abnormal shape
Face	Characteristic facies, e.g. Down's syndrome Cleft lip Asymmetry
Mouth	Cleft lip Teeth Cysts Cleft palate Macroglossia
Ears	Skin creases, e.g. Beckwith–Wiedemann syndrome Deformity/absence Pre-auricular skin tags
Eyes	Absence Asymmetry Absent red reflexes Corneal opacities Coloboma
Neck	Extra skin folds Asymmetry Dimples Swelling
Hands and feet	Asymmetry/absence Swelling
Arms and legs	Asymmetry/absence
Digits	Too few/too many Appearance of nails Appearance of digits

Head

Shape

The shape of the head can provide useful information, e.g. certain syndromes or sequences of abnormal development result in an abnormally shaped head, as does premature closure of certain sutures (craniosynostosis). A less worrying cause of asymmetry is a postural deformity acquired *in utero*; this will resolve with time.

TABLE 5.6 Final part of the examination

Part of body/system	Abnormalities to look out for
Skin	Aplasia cutis Birth marks Cuts or bruises Pigmentation
Chest	Shape Nipple position and number
Cardiovascular system	Heart position Heaves and thrills Heart sounds and murmurs (5 spots) Peripheral pulses
Respiratory system	Respiratory effort Breath sounds
Abdomen	Distension/shape Organomegaly Tenderness
Umbilicus	Condition of cord Condition of surrounding skin
Male genitalia	Testes Shape and size of penis Position of meatus Urine stream
Female genitalia	Appearance Withdrawal bleeding
Anus	Patency Position Passage of meconium
Groin	Swelling
Hips	Stability
Spine	Deformity Overlying marks/defects
Central nervous system	Symmetry of reflexes Appropriateness of reflexes Ability to suck Tone Posture
Size	Weight Length Head circumference

Fontanelles and sutures (Figure 5.1)

Fontanelles are areas where at least three bony plates of the skull meet. They can be felt as soft spots on the head. The posterior fontanelle normally measures less than 0.5 cm at birth and closes shortly after it. The anterior fontanelle normally measures 1–5 cm in diameter at birth and does not close until 18 months of age. The anterior fontanelle at rest should neither bulge nor be sunken. It will bulge as the baby cries.

Sutures are the gaps between two bony plates of the skull. At birth the sutures may be easily palpable, but the bone edges are not widely separated. Premature fusion of a suture may be palpable as a prominent edge, but beware, because overriding sutures can often be felt following delivery, but they will resolve with time.

Size

The occipitofrontal head circumference is measured by placing a tape measure around the head to encircle the occiput, the parietal bones and the forehead (1 cm above the nasal bridge), i.e. the largest circumference. This measurement should be repeated three times and the greatest measurement of the three is taken as being correct. There are centile charts available that take into account the baby's sex and gestation, but if these are not available the normal range for a term baby is between 32 and 37 cm.

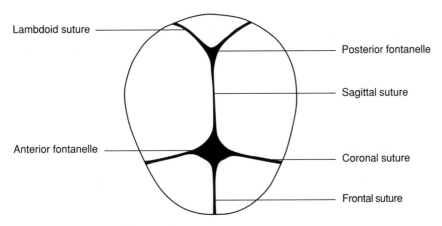

FIGURE 5.1 Fontanelles and sutures

Face

The face can be analysed as a whole, or its components can be scrutinised individually (see below). The overall appearance of the face can be characteristic in certain syndromes, e.g. Down's syndrome, Edward's syndrome (see Chapter 6). Individual features in isolation do not necessarily indicate a syndrome, but in combination with other features they make a syndrome more likely. The practitioner should endeavour to see both the parents before commenting on abnormal facies, as they may simply be familial.

It is also important to look at the symmetry of the face. Asymmetry may result from abnormalities of development of individual components, postural deformities or syndromes, e.g. hemihypertrophy, Goldenhar's syndrome (see Chapter 6).

Skin

The skin of the face should be uniformly pink in colour and free from swellings, abrasions and lesions.

Nose

Babies are nasal breathers. The nose is often squashed *in utero* or during the time of delivery, or it may not be completely patent. Occluding each nostril in turn will check for patency of the opposite nostril.

Lips

External abnormalities of the lips are usually obvious, but internal abnormalities are not necessarily so. Internal examination may require the use of a spatula and a light source.

Mouth

Alveolar ridges (gums)

These must be inspected for cysts, clefts and neonatal teeth.

Tongue

Careful examination should reveal cysts or dimples. The tongue size should also be noted and the underside of the tongue should be inspected along with the floor of the mouth.

Palate

This should be inspected carefully to exclude the presence of a cleft palate. It is not sufficient just to palpate the palate as clefts of the soft palate may be missed in this way.

Ears

These should be looked at for size, shape, position, abnormalities, e.g. skin creases, and surrounding anomalies, e.g. dimples and skin tags. Peculiarities should be discussed with the parents, for they may be familial.

Eyes

The practitioner must be familiar with the normal anatomy of the eye prior to its examination (Figure 5.2). Check carefully to make sure that there are two of them. Look at their size, their position (including

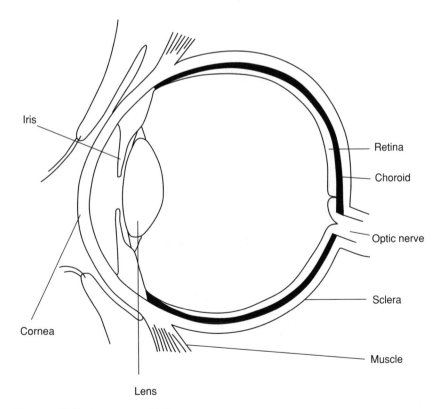

FIGURE 5.2 Anatomy of the eye

distance of separation), the features around them (epicanthic folds, eyelids and eyebrows) and the slant of the palpebral fissures (Figure 5.3).

The sclera are normally white. A yellow discoloration occurs with jaundice; the sclera may be blue in a baby with osteogenesis imperfecta (brittle bone disease), and it is relatively common for there to be haemorrhages after delivery. The iris of a baby is normally blue. It should be perfectly circular with a round opening (the pupil) in the centre. It usually appears to have fibres radiating out from the centre. The presence of white spots on the iris may be significant and therefore may require further detailed examination by an ophthalmologist. The cornea and lens should be clear. Opacification may be secondary to congenital glaucoma, in which there is obstruction to the drainage of the eye, or a cataract (opacification of the lens). You should be able to elicit a red reflex by illuminating the eye with the ophthalmoscope set at +10 dioptres and held 15–20 cm from the eye. Failure to do so may be because of cataracts or a retinoblastoma (a tumour of the retina).

Cataracts can be seen with the naked eye by shining a bright light tangentially. If there is any doubt, more detailed examination should be undertaken.

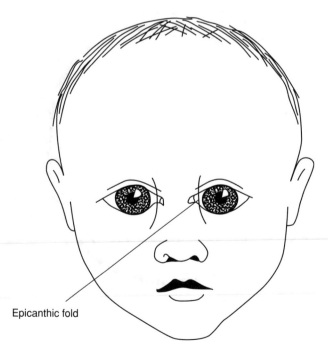

Epicanthic fold

FIGURE 5.3 Epicanthic folds

Neck

The neck may be shortened or webbed, or there may be restriction of the range of movement (congenital torticollis). The neck should have no abnormal swellings or dimples.

The clavicles should be examined for fractures, especially if there is any history of shoulder dystocia or any suggestion of an Erb's palsy.

Limbs

These should be of normal proportions, symmetrical and normally formed.

Hands and feet

The hands and feet are not normally puffy. They should be positioned in line with the limbs and be symmetrical to each other. There are usually multiple palmar creases and creases the length of the sole of the foot in the term baby.

Digits

Count the number of digits on each hand and foot. The digits should not be fused, shortened or abnormally shaped. The nails should be perfectly formed.

Chest

The chest should be symmetrical and there should only be two nipples, each situated just lateral to the midclavicular line, one on each side.

Cardiovascular system

When we refer to the cardiovascular system, we do not refer solely to the heart, although for most parents this seems to be the most important part of that system. In our examination of the cardiovascular system, the following should be considered:

- heart rate
- heart rhythm
- heart position

- pulse volume
- heart noises (see later and Chapter 6)

In addition, the effort of the heart and its effect on other tissues, e.g. liver, oxygenation, etc. should be noted.

Congenital heart disease is said to have an incidence of 8:1000 live births (Haworth and Bull 1993). In order to be able to understand congenital heart disease, knowledge of the heart, its connections and the changes that occur after delivery is necessary.

From fetal to neonatal heart

In utero, the fetal heart and its connections allow the passage of oxygen-rich blood from the placenta via the right side of the heart and pulmonary artery to the aorta, almost bypassing the lungs (Figure 5.4).

After delivery, the supply of oxygen-rich blood from the placenta stops and the right side of the heart is supplied with oxygen-poor blood from the body. The lungs are inflated and the pressure required to perfuse the lungs falls. This results in the preferential perfusion of the lungs with this oxygen-poor blood. This blood becomes oxygenated in the lungs and is then returned to the left side of the heart to be distributed to the body via the aorta. The increased oxygen content of the blood causes the ductus arteriosus to close and the relatively higher pressure on the left side of the heart causes the foramen ovale to close, resulting in the blood in the two sides of the heart being separated (Figure 5.5). These changes do not occur instantly: there is a gradual transition from one state to the other.

In the presence of a heart anomaly, the clinical findings and their time of onset are determined by the nature of the anomaly and the speed with which the changes (described above) occur. This means that not all heart anomalies will be detectable during the course of the neonatal examination.

Colour

Most babies are pink, although some babies exhibit acrocyanosis (cyanosis of the peripheries) without significance. Central cyanosis is, however, pathological. Cyanosis occurs when blood becomes desaturated, i.e. carries less oxygen. Not all babies with congenital heart disease are cyanosed. When cyanosis is present, it can result from three different mechanisms:

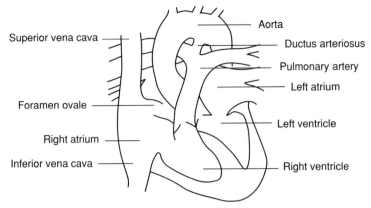

FIGURE 5.4 The fetal heart

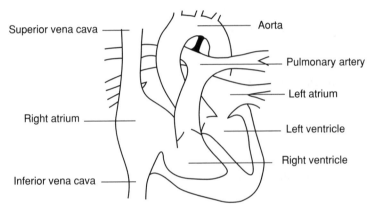

FIGURE 5.5 The neonatal heart and its connections

- low pulmonary blood flow
- transposition streaming
- complete intracardiac mixing.

LOW PULMONARY BLOOD FLOW

Low pulmonary blood flow results from obstruction to blood leaving the right side of the heart (right outflow obstruction). While the ductus arteriosus is patent, the lungs may be perfused by blood from the left side of the heart, but once the ductus closes pulmonary blood flow is reduced. The neonate then becomes cyanosed, but not usually breathless. In the absence of any septal defects, left ventricular output may be reduced, but if there is an accompanying septal defect, right-to-left shunting may occur and sustain left ventricular output. Examples of this include critical pulmonary stenosis, subvalvular obstruction as occurs in Fallot's tetralogy and, as an extreme case, pulmonary atresia (see Chapter 6).

TRANSPOSITION STREAMING

Transposition streaming is a term used to describe the unfavourable streaming of desaturated blood from the vena cava into the aorta. While the ductus arteriosus is patent, mixing of saturated with desaturated blood is possible. Once the ductus closes, unless there is an accompanying septal defect, mixing cannot occur and the neonate develops two separate circulations. One circulation carries saturated blood from the lungs to the heart and back again, and the other carries desaturated blood from the body to the heart and back again. The neonate then becomes cyanosed, but breathlessness does not develop unless there is an accompanying septal defect.

COMPLETE INTRACARDIAC MIXING

Complete intracardiac mixing can occur at one of three levels:

- atrial, e.g. unobstructed total anomalous pulmonary venous drainage;
- ventricular, e.g. univentricular heart; and
- great arteries, e.g. truncus arteriosus.

The degree of cyanosis depends on the relative amounts of saturated (well oxygenated) and desaturated (poorly oxygenated) blood in the mixture and this in turn is dictated by the pulmonary blood flow, i.e. reduced pulmonary blood flow results in reduced saturated blood. Whether the neonate is breathless is also determined by the amount of pulmonary blood flow.

Heart rate and rhythm

The normal resting heart rate of a term neonate is approximately 90–140 beats per minute and the rhythm is normally regular. Minor variations in regularity can occur as a result of varying blood flow through the lungs with each breath.

Femoral pulses/pulse volume

Femoral pulses should be easily palpable in the groin of the neonate. Comparison of the femoral pulse volume with the brachial pulse volume (palpable in the antecubital fossa) may give further useful information, as may comparison of the right brachial pulse volume with the left brachial pulse volume. This part of the examination is best deferred until the groin is examined, but must not be forgotten.

Apical impulse

The apical impulse is normally palpable in the midclavicular line in the fifth intercostal space. It can give useful information as to the position of the heart.

Heaves/thrills

A heave is the term used to describe a diffuse impulse. A heave is best detected by placing the medial side of the hand on the chest wall in the region of the sternum (see Figure 5.6) and applying light pressure. The hand will be felt to lift very slightly with each cardiac impulse.

A thrill represents a murmur that is loud enough to be palpable. A thrill may feel like a cat purring or like a bluebottle trapped in the hand. Thrills are best appreciated during the expiratory phase of respiration, but, for obvious reasons, this is not always practical in a neonate.

Heart sounds

Normally, only two heart sounds will be audible. Traditionally, the first heart sound is said to sound like 'lub' and the second to sound like 'dub'. The first heart sound (best heard at the apex) represents the closure of the mitral and tricuspid valves. The second heart sound (best heard at the second intercostal space) is actually split. The first component represents closure of the aortic valve and the second represents closure of the pulmonary valve. The split between these components normally becomes more evident during the inspiratory phase of respiration, but in a neonate, with a relatively rapid heart rate, the split is difficult to detect. Heart sounds are summarised in Table 5.7.

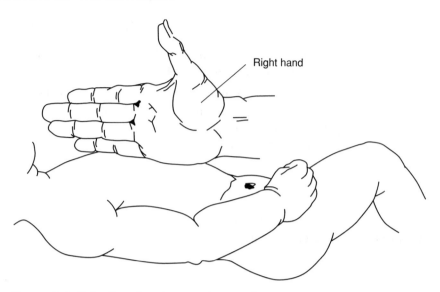

Right hand

FIGURE 5.6 Palpating the chest to detect a heave

TABLE 5.7 Audible heart sounds

Heart sound	Where	What
First	Apex	Closure of mitral and tricuspid valves
Second	Second intercostal space	Closure of aortic and pulmonary valves

The human ear cannot normally detect third and fourth heart sounds. The third heart sound represents ventricular filling that starts as soon as the mitral and tricuspid valves open, and the fourth heart sound represents ventricular filling that occurs in response to contraction of the atria.

Murmurs

A murmur is an additional noise heard during the cardiac cycle. It is usually audible as a soft whooshing noise. In order to be able to interpret the relevance of a murmur, knowledge of the position of the structures of the heart in relation to the surface markings of the chest (see Figure 5.7) is needed.

It is good practice to listen to at least **five** areas of the chest wall to exclude the presence of a heart murmur; these are:

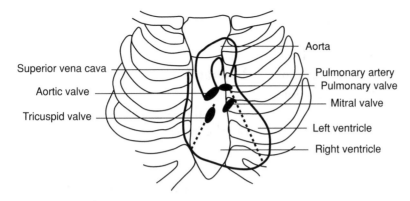

Figure 5.7 Position of the structures of the heart in relation to the surface markings of the chest

1 the apex (mitral area);
2 lower left sternal edge, at the fourth intercostal space (tricuspid area);
3 left of the sternum in the second intercostal space (pulmonary area);
4 right of the sternum in the second intercostal space (aortic area); and
5 midscapular area, posteriorly (coarctation area).

When listening for a murmur, it is useful to palpate the brachial pulse simultaneously in order to determine whether a murmur is systolic or diastolic in timing and at what point in the cycle it occurs. If it occurs during the systolic phase of the cardiac cycle it occurs between the 'lub' and the 'dub' (see heart sounds p. 77). A diastolic murmur is audible between the 'dub' and the next 'lub' of the heart sounds.

- *An ejection systolic murmur* starts just after the onset of systole and is maximal halfway through it.
- *A pansystolic murmur* extends throughout systole, starting at the same time as the first heart sound and is accentuated slightly in mid-systole. It may extend slightly into diastole.
- *An early diastolic murmur* starts early on in diastole and is decrescendo.
- *A mid-diastolic murmur* starts later in diastole and is loudest in mid-diastole.
- *A presystolic murmur* occurs late in diastole.

The loudness of the murmur, which is graded from one to six, should also be documented as follows:

Grade 1   Just audible with the patient's breath held
Grade 2   Quiet
Grade 3   Moderately loud
Grade 4   Accompanied by a thrill
Grade 5   Very loud
Grade 6   Audible without a stethoscope and with the
            head away from the chest

It is also not sufficient to assume that the murmur is audible only at that one position; it should also be documented whether the murmur radiates anywhere else.

Start by listening at the apex with the bell of the stethoscope. The diastolic murmur best heard at the **apex** with the bell of the stethoscope is that of mitral stenosis. Next, listen over the lower left sternal edge (**tricuspid area**) with the diaphragm. Murmurs audible in this area, with the diaphragm, include the diastolic murmurs of aortic and pulmonary incompetence and tricuspid stenosis, and the systolic murmur of tricuspid incompetence. Next, listen over the second left intercostal space (**pulmonary area**) with the diaphragm. The murmur best heard in this area with the diaphragm is the systolic murmur of pulmonary stenosis. Next, listen over the second right intercostal space (**aortic area**) with the diaphragm to hear the systolic murmur of aortic stenosis. Finally, listen in the mid-scapular area with the diaphragm for the systolic murmur of a coarctation. This examination is summarised in Table 5.8.

Liver size

The liver edge in a neonate is usually palpable anything up to 1 cm below the costal margin. It may be enlarged in the presence of heart failure.

Lung fields

When listening to the lungs there are usually only breath sounds audible, i.e. the lung fields are usually clear. Fine crackles may be audible in the presence of heart failure.

TABLE 5.8 Examination of the heart

Where	How	What
Apex	Bell	Diastolic murmur: mitral stenosis
Lower left sternal edge	Diaphragm	Diastolic murmur: aortic and pulmonary incompetence
		Diastolic murmur: tricuspid stenosis
		Systolic murmur: tricuspid incompetence
		Pansystolic murmur: ventricular septal defect
Second left intercostal space	Diaphragm	Systolic murmur: pulmonary stenosis
Second right intercostal space	Diaphragm	Systolic murmur: aortic stenosis
		Systolic/pansystolic murmur: patent ductus arteriosus
Midscapular	Diaphragm	Systolic murmur: coarctation

Note
Absence of a heart murmur does not totally exclude a major cardiac anomaly.

Respiratory system

Colour

Not all babies with respiratory disease are cyanosed. Cyanosis can be a relatively late feature and is often preceded by pallor.

Respiratory effort

The neonate usually breathes without much effort. Respirations are usually quiet, chest movement is usually symmetrical and there is not normally any recession or use of accessory muscles for respiration.

Respiratory noises

A well baby normally breathes relatively quietly. Grunting is a term used to describe a noise that occurs when the neonate attempts to exhale against a partially closed glottis in an effort to avoid collapse of the alveoli. It may only be present when the neonate is disturbed or it may be present with every breath and be accompanied by other symptoms of respiratory disease.

Respiratory rate

Most neonates breathe around 40–60 breaths per minute. Their pattern of breathing is usually reasonably regular, but it is known for them sometimes to have periods of up to 10 seconds when they appear not to breathe. Rapid breathing (tachypnoea), erratic breathing or failure to breathe (apnoea) are all abnormal.

Air entry

When listening to the lungs there are usually only breath sounds audible, i.e. the lung fields are usually clear. Air entry is usually symmetrical, but because of the relatively close proximity of the larger airways to the chest wall, the breath sounds may sound bronchial in nature (like those heard over the throat or over a patch of pneumonia). This, combined with the relatively small surface area of the neonate's chest, makes it more difficult to differentiate between normal lung tissue and pneumonia in the neonate by auscultation alone. Crackles (crepitations) may indicate underlying infection, retained secretions, aspiration or heart failure. Wheeze (rhonchi) and stridor (a sound made during expiration) occur with airway obstruction.

Percussion note

The percussion note over the lungs is usually resonant. Pneumonia will give a dull percussion note and a pneumothorax will give a hyper-resonant note.

Abdomen

Colour

Most babies' abdomens are pink. Deviation from pink may indicate underlying pathology, e.g. a dusky colour may indicate necrotic bowel, redness may indicate inflamed bowel and a periumbilical flare may indicate local infection.

Shape

The abdomen is normally neither distended nor scaphoid (sunken). The shape can change depending on whether the baby has recently been fed, whether he is crying, whether the bladder is full or whether the baby has or is about to open his bowels. Extremes of shape can indicate underlying pathology, e.g. bowel obstruction, diaphragmatic hernia, etc.

Enlarged organs (organomegaly) and masses

In a baby, the pelvis is relatively shallow and the diaphragm is not as deep. This means that some of the organs, which would not normally be easily palpable in an adult, become easily palpable if enlarged. The other two differences between a baby and an adult are:

1 Babies are not generally obese. This makes palpation of organs and masses easier.
2 The spleen enlarges downwards rather than across and downwards (Figure 5.8).

Percussion of the abdomen may provide useful information; it can usually differentiate solid or fluid-filled masses from a gas-filled bowel.

Palpation of the abdomen is best performed by approaching from the right-hand side of the baby. The right hand is gently placed on the abdomen and superficial palpation is performed in all four corners and centrally. Once the baby is used to this, deeper palpation may be attempted. This is done by lying the index and middle fingers across the abdomen and gently but firmly stroking them up the abdominal wall, or by gently pushing the tips of the same two fingers in the direction of the head away from the rest of the hand.

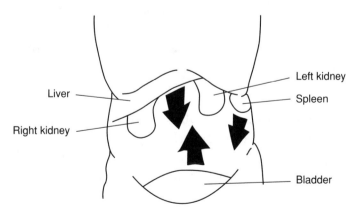

FIGURE 5.8 Position of the abdominal organs and their direction of enlargement in a neonate

PALPATION OF THE LIVER EDGE

Start in the lower right quadrant and work slowly upwards towards the right subcostal area. The procedure should be repeated centrally as the left lobe of the liver may be enlarged independently. A liver edge is normally palpable anything up to 1 cm below the costal margin. An edge palpable at greater than 1 cm may be abnormal.

PALPATION OF THE SPLEEN

Start in the lower left quadrant and work slowly upwards. The spleen can be readily differentiated from the left kidney as it has a notch, which is relatively easily palpable, and it moves with respirations.

PALPATION OF THE KIDNEYS

Place the left hand on the left loin and the fingers of the right hand on the front of the abdomen overlying the left hand. Gently push the left hand forward towards the right hand. Repeat this procedure on the right-hand side to palpate the right kidney. The right kidney may just be palpable, for it tends to lie lower down on the posterior abdominal wall owing to the presence of the liver on the same side. The left is often impalpable.

PALPATION OF THE BLADDER

The bladder is often felt as a 'fullness' rising up from the pelvis.

PALPATION OF MASSES

As with an intra-abdominal organ, any abdominal mass must be examined by means of inspection, palpation, percussion and even auscultation in order to have any idea of its origin. Knowledge of the stages of development of the contents of the abdomen is valuable as it may assist the identification of a mass, but this is beyond the scope of this book.

TENDERNESS

It is sometimes difficult to tell whether a baby has tenderness or not. Tenderness usually indicates underlying pathology, but it may only be indicated by a rigid abdomen, a crying baby or a baby who draws his knees up – all signs that may be found under other circumstances.

Umbilicus

Condition of cord

The size of the cord may give clues about the intrauterine growth of the baby – heavier babies tend to have cords with more Wharton's jelly, whereas growth-retarded babies often have thin cords.

As the cord separates, it may become moist and smell. Simple cord care with an alcohol swab will help keep it dry until separation occurs.

Condition of surrounding skin

Around the time of separation, there is often a small degree of redness surrounding the attachment of the cord. This is usually unimportant, but if it begins to spread and extend up the abdominal wall it may indicate ascending infection that will require treatment.

Number of vessels in cord

When the cord is severed, it is usually apparent that there are two arteries and one vein. There is an association of renal anomalies with cords with only one artery, but some clinicians consider this association is not sufficiently strong to justify further investigations.

Male genitalia

Scrotum

The scrotum may be relatively smooth or have a rugged appearance. It may have a midline ridge. A large scrotum may be the result of a hydrocele. If this is the case, it will transilluminate when a bright light is placed next to it in a darkened room. Occasionally, the scrotum develops as a bifid structure; the baby should be examined carefully to confirm that there are testes present in each half of it and that the rest of the genitalia are normal.

Pigmentation of the scrotum is common in babies born to parents who are not white, but it may be an early finding in congenital adrenal hyperplasia. Discoloration of the scrotum occurs with a neonatal torsion of the testis; the testicle is usually painful in this condition.

Testes

The scrotum is usually home to two testicles, which can be felt as two distinct entities, one in each side of the scrotum. Each testicle is approximately 1–1.5 cm diameter, but may feel larger if there is an accompanying hydrocele. In the absence of one testicle, the groin on the side of the absent testicle should be carefully palpated as the testicle may not have completed its descent from the posterior abdominal wall. It is also worthwhile palpating just below the groin as the testicle may have descended abnormally to that area. Absence of both testicles should alert the practitioner to the fact that the baby's sex may be indeterminate. This will necessitate careful examination of the baby and further investigations.

Penis

The size of the penis at birth varies considerably, but if there are concerns about size there are centile charts for stretched penile length. There is little variation in shape of the penis, but abnormalities can occur. The skin on the underside of the penis can be tethered to the scrotum (chordee). The foreskin may be hooded in appearance and this may or may not be associated with an abnormally placed meatus (hypospadias). A malpositioned meatus may be associated with abnormalities of the urethra and kidneys and may result in a poor urinary stream.

Female genitalia

Labia

As with the scrotum in the male baby, the appearance and colour of the labia are important things to note. Large labia may alert the practitioner to the fact that she is dealing with a baby of indeterminate sex and that there may be testes within them. They may also appear large in small for dates and preterm babies.

Pigmentation of the labia is common in babies born to parents who are not white, but it may also be an early finding in congenital adrenal hyperplasia.

Vagina

The hymen may cover the vaginal orifice, and may be imperforate in some babies. Sometimes, vaginal skin tags are visible and may appear large in comparison with the labia. Shortly after birth, some babies suffer withdrawal bleeding and it is not uncommon for this to continue for several days.

Clitoris

The clitoris may seem quite large in small for dates and preterm babies, but its size must be assessed in comparison with its associated structures. If it is felt that it is inordinately large then the baby should be examined carefully to exclude an indeterminate sex.

Meatus

The position of the urinary meatus is a little more difficult to see in a female baby, but should be positioned between the clitoris and the vaginal orifice and the urinary stream should be good.

Anus

Patency

The patency of the anus is not always easy to assess. Even babies who have clearly been documented as having passed meconium within hours of birth have sometimes gone on to develop problems associated with patency because of a slightly malpositioned anus. It is important to take note of whether or not a baby has passed meconium, allowing for the fact that this may be delayed if the baby passed meconium *in utero*.

Position

The position of the anus in relation to the other perineal structures may alert the practitioner to potential problems. An anteriorly placed anus may be associated with problems, e.g. malformation of the rectum, constipation in later life, etc.

The practitioner should also look carefully for evidence of leakage of meconium from sites other than the anus. Never assume that the meconium at the tip of the urinary meatus or covering the vaginal orifice is from the anus; it may be coming from a fistula (an abnormal connection with the rectum).

Groin

Perhaps one of the important things to determine here, is whether or not the femoral pulses are palpable. The significance of this finding has been discussed in the cardiovascular section.

Swellings in the groin are not uncommon. They may be mal-descended testes or hydroceles in the male baby, malpositioned ovaries in the female baby or herniae or vascular anomalies in either.

Hips

The hips should appear symmetrical; this includes the skin creases on the back of the legs. They should also have a good range of movement, being fully abductable with no resistance to movement. Performing two manoeuvres should check the stability of the hips.

Ortolani's manoeuvre

If performed correctly Ortolani's manoeuvre will detect a congenitally dislocated hip. The baby should be placed on his back on a firm flat surface. The legs are held with the hips and the knees flexed at right angles. The easiest way to do this is to hold the palm of the hand against the baby's shin, the thumb of the hand on the inside of the baby's thigh and the middle finger overlying the greater trochanter of the femur. The hips are slowly abducted from the midline position, through 90° while pushing forwards with the middle finger. A dislocated hip will clunk back into the acetabulum as this manoeuvre is performed. Failure to abduct the hips fully is suggestive of congenital dislocation, but not confirmatory. A click may be felt as a result of laxity of the ligaments of the hip or it may originate from the knee.

Barlow's manoeuvre

If performed correctly Barlow's manoeuvre will identify an easily dislocatable hip. With the legs held as for Ortolani's manoeuvre, pressure is applied to the front of the knee, forcing the femur to slide backwards. An unstable hip will dislocate out of the acetabulum. Performing Ortolani's manoeuvre can then relocate it.

If a dislocated or dislocatable hip is detected, the two manoeuvres should not be repeated, as there is a risk that the femoral head may suffer avascular necrosis. It should also be noted that it is practice in some maternity units to routinely scan the hips of breech babies.

Spine

The spine is best examined by placing the baby face down, with its abdomen and chest in the palm of one hand. The skin overlying the spine should be inspected, as an overlying abnormality of skin, e.g. a tuft of hair, a pit or a birthmark may be an indication of an underlying abnormality.

Deformity can be easily seen, but it is also worthwhile feeling along the length of the spine to ensure that it runs a straight course.

Central nervous system

Behaviour

Take note of the everyday behaviour of the baby; a quiet baby may have a neurological problem, as may an irritable baby. Observe the baby's reaction to external stimuli; does he startle to loud noise, quieten to the spoken word, close the eyes in response to bright light, cry when undressed and cry when a feed is due.

Cry

In order to appreciate an abnormal cry the practitioner has to be familiar with what a normal cry sounds like. The best way to do this is to spend time on a postnatal ward listening to babies cry.

Movement

Movement should be symmetrical, inasmuch as both arms and legs should move equally and the muscles of the face should produce symmetrical expressions. Asymmetrical movement may indicate injury to nerve(s), e.g. Erb's palsy, injury to bone, e.g. fracture of the clavicle or neurological abnormality, e.g. Möebius' syndrome (see Chapter 6).

Babies often appear to be jittery when they move. This probably represents an exaggerated response to movement. We forget that as adults we have had years to perfect our movements and that these movements have taken place in a free environment. Before delivery, babies are restricted by the confines of the uterus. They have never had to rely on the mechanisms that make our movements so precise. When they are born and those confines disappear, they suddenly have freedom of movement, but not precision of movement, which results in them 'overshooting their mark' and appearing jittery. It is worth remembering that a baby can also be jittery as a result of hypoglycaemia, hypocalcaemia, infection or neurological problems.

Fits are not common in babies, but when they do occur they are often more subtle than those seen in adults and older children. They may be rhythmical jerking movements or they may be merely repetitive cycling or sucking movements, both of which can be subtle.

Posture and tone

When first born, a baby will often adopt the position he was in *in utero*. Soon after birth he begins to adopt a flexed/curled position. This change takes longer to achieve in the preterm baby, but there are charts available for assessment of posture with relation to gestational age. A baby with reduced tone (hypotonic) may fail to flex, whereas a baby with increased tone (hypertonia) may adopt an extended position. Both posture and tone are controlled by the central nervous system, although neuromuscular problems will also affect both.

Hypotonia can be detected by supporting the baby by placing the practitioner's hands, one under each axilla. A baby with normal tone will remain supported, but a baby with central hypotonia will 'slip' through the hands of the practitioner. Central hypotonia can be confirmed by lying the baby face down, with its abdomen and chest in the palm of one of the practitioner's hands. A baby with normal tone will attempt to raise the head and the legs, but a baby with hypotonia will lie limply in the practitioner's hand like a rag doll.

Reflexes

Perhaps the most important thing to take note of when assessing neonatal reflexes is whether or not they are symmetrical. The interpretation of neonatal reflexes must take place with the baby in a neutral (midline) position, as rotation of the head to one or other side during assessment can influence the findings.

The reflexes used to assess the neonate differ slightly from those used to assess older children and adults. In addition to the knee, ankle and biceps reflexes, which should be present, symmetrical and not exaggerated, there are also the Moro reflex, the stepping reflex, the rooting reflex, suck reflex and the palmar and plantar grasp reflexes.

- *The Moro reflex* is elicited by taking the baby in both hands, the head being supported by one hand and the buttocks by the other. With the baby's head in a midline position, the hand supporting it is quickly dropped to a position approximately 10 cm below its original supporting position, and the head is caught by the hand in its new position. In response, the baby will throw out both arms and legs symmetrically.
- *The stepping reflex* can be elicited by holding the baby under the shoulders with both hands. The baby's shin is placed in contact with the side of the cot and the baby will perform a stepping/climbing manoeuvre. This is repeated for the other leg.
- *The rooting reflex* is elicited by gently stroking the skin of the baby's cheek. He will turn the head towards the side that is being stimulated.
- *The suck reflex* is elicited by placing the practitioner's clean little finger in the baby's mouth. The baby will suck on the finger as it would on a nipple or teat. Failure of the baby to suck may indicate underlying neurological damage, but before jumping to any such conclusion, it is worth noting whether the baby has recently been fed and whether the baby is sleepy.
- *Palmar grasp reflex* is elicited by placing the practitioner's little finger into the palm of the baby. The baby's hand will grasp the practitioner's finger. Care should be taken not to touch the back of the hand at the same time as the finger is placed in contact with the palm as this can result in conflicting sensory information being presented to the neurones and an uninterpretable result being obtained.
- *Plantar grasp reflex* is elicited by touching the sole of the baby's foot with the practitioner's little finger. The baby's toes will flex towards the practitioner's finger. Care should be taken not to touch the dorsum of the foot at the same time as the finger makes contact with the sole as this can result in conflicting information being relayed to the neurones and an uninterpretable result being obtained.

Assessment of intrauterine growth

Once this is complete, all that remains is to measure the baby's length and refer to the appropriate centile chart to check on size. Do not forget to check the birth weight and occipitofrontal head circumference (see earlier) at the same time.

Measurement of length can be a difficult procedure to perform correctly and requires the assistance of a second person and suitable equipment. Most hospitals have a stadiometer, which is a device for correctly measuring length; it is not sufficient to use a tape measure if an accurate assessment of length is required. The baby is placed on the stadiometer with his head firmly against the top end. The baby is then carefully stretched and the mobile bar is brought up to make contact with the flat of the baby's foot. The baby must be lying flat, with the head in contact with the top end of the stadiometer and the pelvis in a neutral position, i.e. not tilted. The measurement is then read off the scale at the side of the stadiometer.

Use of centile charts is not difficult, but there is one peculiarity in their use. Although centile charts clearly have the weeks of gestation marked on their *x*-axis, a baby born at 36 weeks' gestation and above always has its birth measurements plotted as though it had been born at 40 weeks' gestation because it is deemed to be full-term. Always make sure you have referred to the correct centile chart for the baby's sex and be aware that there are alternative centile charts for conditions such as Turner's syndrome and Down's syndrome, even though your hospital or practice may not routinely stock them.

Check list

When the examination is complete, the practitioner must make sure that the following are undertaken:

1 document findings (normal or abnormal)
2 inform the parents of any findings (normal or abnormal)
3 inform the paediatrician who is responsible for the care of the baby
4 inform the staff caring for the baby and parent(s)
5 document who has been informed and when
6 document any action(s) taken
7 provide the parents with the opportunity to ask further questions.

Step 4: explanation to the parent(s)

It is best practice to talk through the examination with the parent(s) while it is happening, so those questions that arise can be addressed in context. For example, as you are examining the baby's spine you can verbalize what you are expecting to find, 'I am feeling to see whether his backbone is in line and that there are no unusual lumps or dimples – and look, his spine is beautifully in line.' It may seem obvious to give a running commentary as you go along; however, an examiner's careful concentration can easily be misinterpreted for concern, and therefore inadvertently raise anxiety levels in the parent(s). If you engage in conversation, it also makes it easier for concerns to be raised. If you conduct the examination in silence, parent(s) may be afraid to interrupt your concentration and therefore they may not ask questions. It is also an opportunity to confirm the normality of features that may be alarming to the new mother or father, such as the shape of the baby's head after delivery or the appearance of the navel. Any abnormal finding must be conveyed to the parent(s) and this issue is discussed in Chapter 6.

Step 5: documentation

The printed documentation of each trust will have a section within the baby notes that the practitioner must complete after the examination of the newborn. It usually comprises a checklist against which you can record your findings. Completing the records in view of the parent(s) provides another opportunity for reassuring the parents that you are satisfied that the baby appears well. Contemporaneous record keeping also helps avoid the potential errors of recall that may occur if records are completed some time after the event.

We have a professional duty to keep clear and accurate records of our observations and actions (UKCC 1998b) and this issue is discussed in detail in Chapter 7 under the section 'Achieving and maintaining best practice'.

The next chapter considers the identification of abnormal findings and how the practitioner examining the newborn infant should manage such discoveries.

Chapter 6

Abnormal findings and congenital abnormalities

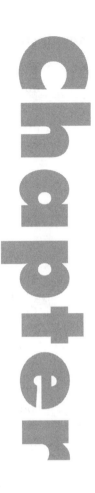

- Introduction
- Abnormal findings
- Specific abnormalities
- Specific syndromes
- Summary

Introduction

The aim of this chapter is to consider abnormalities that may be found during the first examination of the neonate and make suggestions regarding their appropriate management. It is important that the practitioner is able to recognise the significance of an abnormal finding and to differentiate between those that require:

- immediate medical attention
- referral to a paediatrician for follow-up
- explanation or reassurance by the practitioner.

It is assumed that if an abnormality is discovered it will be discussed with a paediatrician, but the practitioner must be familiar with the local guidelines on investigation and management of individual conditions. The practitioner will also need to be familiar with normal laboratory values for the local hospital.

This chapter is divided into two major sections (abnormal findings and congenital abnormalities). The first section concentrates on individual abnormal findings and their relevance. The second section concentrates on the more common congenital abnormalities. The order of each section is similar to the previous chapter to enable the practitioner to move between chapters and sections in the order that the baby is examined and that abnormalities may be discovered. Whenever an abnormality is detected, the baby should be examined carefully to exclude other abnormalities.

Before embarking on the subject of abnormalities and how to deal with them, there are several important things to remember when examining a baby in the neonatal period. This is an emotional period for both the mother and the father. Everyone expects that their baby will be perfect. To be told that a baby has or may have an abnormality can be devastating to some parents, especially the mother, who for the last 9 months has been the guardian of the baby and feels responsible for its growth and development.

The consequences of an abnormality can often be far reaching not only for the baby and parents, but also for other members of the family. The child may have a reduced life span or may never fulfil his parent's expectations. His parents may have to devote time to unanticipated hospital attendances and allow complete strangers access to their home and family. They may never be able to provide fully for the child's needs, relying on the support and expertise of outside agencies. Siblings may 'lose their place' in the family as their new addition puts increasing demands on time and energy. What was a solid family unit can sometimes be destroyed, resulting in the breakdown of that family.

Because of this, it is important to consider how, when and where parents should be told about an abnormal finding. Ideally, the news should be broken in the presence of support, e.g. with the partner present, in a private place and by someone who can explain in simple terms without being patronising.

However one breaks 'bad news' to parents and family, in their eyes, it will never be done perfectly, but it is up to the bearer of 'bad news' to attempt to do so. It is also important, once the news has been broken, to be available to answer questions and to have some understanding of the agencies which can offer support to the parents and family (see Appendix 1).

Abnormal findings

In Chapter 5 we have already suggested that a great deal of information can be obtained from the maternal notes. Indeed, we may well be alerted to the possibility of an abnormality by just checking the maternal notes (Table 5.2). Even if at first the maternal notes give us no clues about the causes of a problem, it is always worth rechecking them. Some abnormal findings have common causes. In order to avoid repetition throughout the text, Tables 6.1 and 6.2 summarise what investigations and management should be considered if certain common causes are suspected.

Observations

Temperature instability

A temperature of up to 37.2°C is acceptable for a baby in a neonatal unit or a postnatal ward. A temperature of less than 36.5°C is considered to be hypothermic. Occasionally the environmental temperature can influence a baby's temperature, but other causes should be considered (see Table 6.1).

TABLE 6.1 Abnormal observations, possible causes and investigations to consider*

Observations	Abnormality	Causes	Check maternal notes for evidence of	Action/investigation
Temperature	Instability	Intracranial haemorrhage Infection	Antenatal problems Difficult delivery Difficult resuscitation Prolonged rupture of membranes Maternal infection	Consider investigating as for: Infection* Intracranial haemorrhage*
Colour	Peripheral cyanosis	Cold peripheries Congenital heart disease Hypoxia	Difficult delivery Difficult resuscitation	Check baby's temperature Consider investigating as for: Congenital heart disease* Hypoxia*
	Central cyanosis	Congenital heart disease Infection Neuromuscular disease Respiratory disease	Prolonged rupture of membranes Maternal infection	Consider investigating as for: Congenital heart disease* Infection* Neuromuscular disease* Respiratory disease*
	Pallor	Anaemia Hypoxia Infection	Fetal compromise Difficult delivery Difficult resuscitation Prolonged rupture of membranes Maternal infection Maternal antibodies Blood group incompatibility Blood loss	Consider investigating as for: Anaemia* Hypoxia* Infection*
	Plethora	Pyrexia secondary to infection Polycythaemia	Prolonged rupture of membranes Maternal infection	Consider investigating as for: Infection* Polycythaemia*

Sign	Possible causes	Associated factors	Investigation
Jaundice < 48 hours of age	Haemolysis Polycythaemia Infection (including hepatitis) Bruising Galactosaemia	Difficult delivery Prolonged rupture of membranes Maternal infection Maternal antibodies Blood group incompatibility	Bilirubin Consider investigating as for: Galactosaemia* Haemolysis* Infection (including congenital infection)* Polycythaemia*
Jaundice > 48 hours age but < 10 days of age	Physiological Haemolysis Infection Bruising Galactosaemia	Difficult delivery Prolonged rupture of membranes Maternal infection Maternal antibodies Blood group incompatibility	Bilirubin If there is any reason to suspect anything other than physiological jaundice proceed to investigate as for jaundice < 48 hours of age
Behaviour — Abnormal cry	Hypoxia Raised intracranial pressure Infection Neurodevelopmental abnormalities Certain syndromes	Antenatal problems Fetal compromise Difficult delivery Difficult resuscitation Prolonged rupture of membranes Maternal infection	Consider investigating as for: Hypoxia* Infection* Neurodevelopmental abnormalities* Raised intracranial pressure* Syndrome*
Abnormal posture	Hypoxia Raised intracranial pressure Intracranial haemorrhage Infection Neurodevelopmental abnormalities Nerve or bone trauma Hyperbilirubinaemia causing kernicterus	Antenatal problems Fetal compromise Difficult delivery Difficult resuscitation Prolonged rupture of membranes Maternal infection	Bilirubin Consider investigating as for: Hypoxia* Infection* Intracranial haemorrhage* Neurodevelopmental abnormalities* Raised intracranial pressure*

Observations	Abnormality	Causes	Check maternal notes for evidence of	Action/investigation
	Irritable	Hypoxia Raised intracranial pressure Intracranial haemorrhage Infection Neurodevelopmental abnormalities Withdrawal from maternal medication or maternal drugs Pain, e.g. from trauma	Fetal compromise Difficult delivery Difficult resuscitation Maternal medication Maternal drug abuse Prolonged rupture of membranes Maternal infection	Urine toxicology screen on baby and mother Consider investigating as for: Hypoxia* Infection* Intracranial haemorrhage* Neurodevelopmental abnormalities* Raised intracranial pressure*
	Sleepy	Hypoglycaemia Hypermagnesaemia Infection Hyperbilirubinaemia Maternal medication Maternal drug abuse	Maternal medication Maternal drug abuse Maternal glucose intolerance Maternal infection Prolonged rupture of membranes	Blood glucose Bilirubin Magnesium Urine toxicology screen on baby and mother Consider investigating as for: Infection*
Feeding	Vomiting	Hypoxia Raised intracranial pressure Infection Maternal medication or maternal drug abuse Gastrointestinal abnormalities	Fetal compromise Difficult delivery Difficult resuscitation Maternal medication Maternal drug abuse Prolonged rupture of membranes Maternal infection	Urine toxicology screen on baby and mother Blood urea and electrolytes 17-hydroxyprogesterone (at > 48 hours age) Abdominal X-ray with or without contrast Abdominal ultrasound

		Congenital adrenal hyperplasia Galactosaemia		Consider investigating as for: Galactosaemia* Hypoxia* Infection* Raised intracranial pressure*
	Inability to suck or feed	Prematurity Cleft lip or palate Jaundice Neurodevelopmental abnormalities	Prematurity Fetal compromise Difficult delivery Difficult resuscitation	Bilirubin Refer to cleft lip and palate team if either is present Consider referring to speech therapist Consider investigating as for: Neurodevelopmental abnormalities*
Movement	Asymmetry	Ischaemia Haemorrhage Neurodevelopmental abnormalities Nerve or bone injury	Fetal compromise Difficult delivery Difficult resuscitation	Consider investigating as for: Bone injury * Ischaemia* Neurodevelopmental abnormalities*
	Fits	Hypoxia Raised intracranial pressure Haemorrhage Infection Neurodevelopmental abnormalities Hypocalcaemia Hypoglycaemia Maternal medication or maternal drug abuse	Fetal compromise Difficult delivery Difficult resuscitation Maternal medication Maternal drug abuse Prolonged rupture of membranes Maternal infection Glucose intolerance	Calcium Glucose Urine toxicology screen on baby and mother Consider investigating as for: Hypoxia* Infection* Intracranial haemorrhage* Neurodevelopmental abnormalities* Raised intracranial pressure*

Observations	Abnormality	Causes	Check maternal notes for evidence of	Action/investigation
	Jittery	Hypoxia Haemorrhage Infection Neurodevelopmental abnormalities Hypocalcaemia Hypoglycaemia Maternal medication or maternal drug abuse Exaggerated normal response	Fetal compromise Difficult delivery Difficult resuscitation Maternal medication Maternal drug abuse Prolonged rupture of membranes Maternal infection Glucose intolerance	Calcium Glucose Urine toxicology screen on baby and mother Consider investigating as for: Hypoxia* Infection* Intracranial haemorrhage* Neurodevelopmental abnormalities* Raised intracranial pressure*
Chest	Asymmetry	Abnormalities of external structures of the chest pneumothorax Diaphragmatic hernia		Consider investigating as for: Respiratory disease*
	Fast or slow heart rate		Maternal medication Maternal drug abuse Maternal disease, e.g. systemic lupus erythematosus (SLE) or Graves' disease	ECG Thyroid function tests Urine toxicology screen on baby and mother Consider: Discussing with a cardiologist if heart rate > 240 or there is heart block Treating the baby for thyrotoxicosis if present

Finding	Possible cause		Action
Reduced femoral pulse volume or absent femoral pulses	Left ventricular outflow obstruction Infection	Prolonged rupture of membranes Maternal infection	Consider investigating as for: Infection* Congenital heart disease*
Displaced apical impulse	Dextrocardia (heart on the opposite side to normal) Cardiomegaly (enlarged heart) Pneumothorax (air in the thoracic cavity)		Locate the apical impulse by palpation Chest X-ray Consider referring to cardiologist for cardiomegaly or dextrocardia Consider investigating as for: Respiratory disease*
Heave/thrill palpable	Congenital heart disease		Consider investigating as for: Congenital heart disease*
Abnormal heart sounds	Congenital heart disease		Consider investigating as for: Congenital heart disease*
Murmur	Congenital heart disease Anaemia	Maternal antibodies Blood group incompatibility Blood loss	Consider investigating as for: Congenital heart disease* Anaemia*
Recession	Choanal atresia Pneumothorax Infection	Prolonged rupture of membranes Maternal infection	Exclude choanal atresia Consider investigating as for: Respiratory disease* Infection*

Observations	Abnormality	Causes	Check maternal notes for evidence of	Action/investigation
	Grunting	Infection Hypoglycaemia Respiratory distress syndrome Diaphragmatic hernia Pneumothorax Hypoplastic lungs Congenital heart disease	Prematurity Glucose intolerance Prolonged rupture of membranes Maternal infection	Blood sugar Consider investigating as for: Infection* Respiratory disease* Congenital heart disease*
	Tachypnoea	Congenital heart disease Respiratory disease, e.g. respiratory distress syndrome Respiratory abnormality, e.g. diaphragmatic hernia, pneumothorax Metabolic disease Infection	Prematurity Prolonged rupture of membranes Maternal infection	Consider investigating as for: Infection* Respiratory disease* Congenital heart disease* Metabolic disease*
	Irregular/gasping respirations	Hypoxia Congenital heart disease Respiratory disease Respiratory abnormality Maternal opiates Infection Immaturity of the respiratory centre Metabolic disease Neurological disease	Prematurity Fetal compromise Difficult delivery Difficult resuscitation Maternal medication Maternal drug abuse Prolonged rupture of membranes Maternal infection	Urine toxicology screen on baby and mother Consider investigating as for: Hypoxia* Infection* Respiratory disease* Congenital heart disease* Metabolic disease* Neuromuscular disease*

	Causes	Predisposing factors	Investigations
Apnoea	Maternal opiates Infection Immaturity of the respiratory centre Choanal atresia Neurological disease	Prematurity Maternal medication Maternal drug abuse Prolonged rupture of membranes Maternal infection	Exclude choanal atresia Urine toxicology screen on baby and mother Consider investigating as for: Infection* Neuromuscular disease*
Unequal air entry or added sounds	Infection Pneumothorax Heart failure Upper airway obstruction	Prolonged rupture of membranes Maternal infection	Consider investigating as for: Infection* Respiratory disease* Congenital heart disease*
Abdomen			
Discoloration	Infection Bowel obstruction Ischaemic/necrotic bowel	Prolonged rupture of membranes Maternal infection	Abdominal X-ray Consider investigating as for: Infection*
Hepatomegaly	Congenital heart disease Heart failure Congenital infection Metabolic conditions Intrahepatic haemorrhage Vascular anomalies Tumours	Difficult delivery	Glucose Liver function tests Clotting screen (liver ultrasound) Consider investigating as for: Congenital heart disease* Metabolic disease* Congenital infection*
Splenomegaly	Haemolysis Infection Congenital infection Trauma	Difficult delivery Prolonged rupture of membranes Maternal infection Maternal antibodies Blood group incompatibility	Bilirubin (spleen ultrasound) Consider investigating as for: Haemolysis* Infection* Congenital infection*

Observations	Abnormality	Causes	Check maternal notes for evidence of	Action/investigation
Genitalia	Pigment-ation	Ethnic origin Congenital adrenal hyperplasia		Consider checking: Blood electrolyte levels 17-Hydroxyprogesterone levels at 48 hours of age
Central nervous system	Reduced tone or Increased tone	Hypoxia Raised intracranial pressure Intracranial haemorrhage Infection Neurodevelopmental abnormalities	Fetal compromise Difficult delivery Difficult resuscitation Maternal medication Maternal drug abuse Prolonged rupture of membranes Maternal infection	Urine toxicology screen on baby and mother Consider investigating as for: Hypoxia* Infection* Intracranial haemorrhage* Neurodevelopmental abnormalities* Raised intracranial pressure* Syndrome*
	Asymmet-rical reflexes	Hypoxia Raised intracranial pressure Intracranial haemorrhage Neurodevelopmental abnormalities Bone or nerve injury	Fetal compromise Difficult delivery Difficult resuscitation	Urine toxicology screen on baby and mother Consider investigating as for: Hypoxia* Intracranial haemorrhage* Neurodevelopmental abnormalities* Raised intracranial pressure* Bone trauma*

Colour

PERIPHERAL CYANOSIS

This is a blue discoloration of the skin of the hands and feet. It can occur when the baby is cold, but other causes should also be considered (see Table 6.1).

CENTRAL CYANOSIS

In central cyanosis the skin of the hands and feet and the remainder of the body has a blue discoloration, as do the lips and the tongue and the mucous membrane of the mouth. For causes see Table 6.1.

Anaemia reduces the oxygen-carrying capacity of blood and makes cyanosis more difficult to detect as cyanosis only occurs when the amount of desaturated haemoglobin is 5 g per 100 ml.

PALLOR

The skin is pale in colour. For causes see Table 6.1.

PLETHORA

The skin is red or deep pink in colour. For causes see Table 6.1.

JAUNDICE

This is a yellow discoloration of the skin and sclera of the eyes. It occurs when the level of circulating bilirubin becomes elevated. This commonly occurs in the newborn baby about 3 days after delivery as a result of increased red cell breakdown and immaturity of the liver. Jaundice occurring earlier than this, and especially within 24 hours of delivery, usually requires investigation, as does jaundice occurring after 10 days of age. It is also worthwhile considering the possibility of abnormal causes of jaundice in a baby who develops it within the period 3–10 days of age. For causes see Table 6.1.

Behaviour

Abnormal cry

In order to appreciate an abnormal cry the practitioner has to be familiar with what a normal cry sounds like. The best way to do this is to spend time on a postnatal ward listening to the crying of babies. An example of an abnormal cry is a high-pitched cry. For causes see Table 6.1.

TABLE 6.2 Observed conditions with suggested investigations in management

Causes	Check maternal notes for evidence of	Investigation	Possible finding	Management
Anaemia	Blood loss Blood group incompatibility Maternal antibodies	Haemoglobin Direct Coombs test	Low haemoglobin Positive result	Correction of anaemia Monitor bilirubin and haemoglobin Supplemental folic acid
		Blood group (mother and baby) Maternal Kleihauer test	Incompatability Positive with feto-maternal bleed	Check bilirubin
Bone trauma		Radiograph	Fracture/dislocation	Discussion with orthopaedic surgeon
Congenital heart disease		ECG Chest radiograph Hyperoxia test Four-limb blood pressure Echocardiogram	Depends on cardiac lesion	Depends on cardiac lesion, e.g. prostaglandins for duct-dependent lesions
Congenital infection	Maternal infection	Toxoplasma titres Rubella titres Cytomegalovirus (urine culture and throat swab) Hepatitis B and C Platelet count Liver function tests	Result not immediately available May be < 150 May be deranged	

	Predisposing factors	Investigations	Results	Management
Galactosaemia		Urine reducing substances	Positive	Lactose-free milk
		Red blood cell galactose-1-phosphate-uridyl-transferase level	Reduced	
		Liver function tests	May be deranged	
Haemolysis	Blood group incompatibility	Bilirubin	Raised	Phototherapy
	Maternal antibodies	Haemoglobin	Low	Check bilirubin
	Maternal infection	Blood group (mother and baby)	Incompatible	
		Direct Coombs test	Positive	
		Blood film	Abnormal-shaped red cells	
		Red cell enzymes, e.g. glucose-6-phosphate dehydrogenase level	Low levels	
		Consider investigating as for infection		
Hypoxia	Fetal compromise	Arterial blood gas	Hypoxia	Oxygen
	Difficult delivery		Metabolic acidosis (base excess ≥ 10)	Ventilatory support
	Difficult resuscitation			Correction of acidosis

Causes	Check maternal notes for evidence of	Investigation	Possible finding	Management
Infection	Prolonged rupture of membranes Maternal infection	White blood cell count Platelet count Erythrocyte sedimentation rate C-reactive protein Blood culture Surface swabs Urine culture (lumbar puncture)	Raised (refer to laboratory values) < 150 > 10 >10 Result not immediately available	Antibiotics
Intracranial haemorrhage	Antenatal problems Difficult delivery Difficult resuscitation	Cranial ultrasound	May be normal immediately after the haemorrhage	
Ischaemia	Antenatal problems Difficult delivery Difficult resuscitation	Cranial ultrasound (CT scan, MRI scan)		
Metabolic disease		Blood glucose Arterial blood gas	Low May show metabolic acidosis (base excess ≥ 10)	Consider checking insulin and cortisol levels Treat hypoglycaemia Correction of acidosis

Condition	Investigation	Finding	Management
Neurodevelop-mental abnormalities	Urine reducing substance	May be positive	Identify reducing and treat if necessary
	Urine amino and organic acids	May indicate disorder of amino/organic acid pathways	Discuss with consultant with interest in metabolic disorders
	Ammonia	Raised in urea cycle defects	
	Cranial ultrasound scan (CT scan, MRI scan)		Discussion and/or referral to a neurologist or neurosurgeon may be necessary
Neuromuscular disease		Discussion and/or	referral to a neurologist may be necessary
Polycythaemia	Full blood count	Raised haemoglobin Haematocrit > 60%	Dilutional exchange transfusion
	Glucose	Hypoglycaemia	Supplemental glucose
	Bilirubin	Raised	Phototherapy
Raised intra-cranial pressure	Cranial ultrasound scan (CT scan, MRI scan)		Discussion and/or referral to a neurosurgeon may be necessary

Causes	Check maternal notes for evidence of	Investigation	Possible finding	Management
Respiratory disease		Transillumination of the chest	Chest transilluminates with pneumothorax	Thoracocentesis (temporary drainage) Chest drain insertion
		Chest radiograph	May show: Pneumonia Respiratory distress syndrome Pneumothorax	Respiratory support, e.g. oxygen, ventilation Antibiotics for pneumonia Drainage of a symptomatic pneumothorax
		Arterial blood gas	Low $Pa\mathrm{O}_2$ Raised $P\mathrm{CO}_2$ pH < 7.25	
Syndrome	Family history	Chromosome analysis	May be normal	Genetic advice

Abnormal posture

When a baby is first delivered it usually adopts the posture it had *in utero*, e.g. an extended breech baby will attempt to lie with its hips flexed and its feet almost up by its ears. Gradually the baby adopts a flexed posture with elbows, knees and hips flexed. For causes of abnormal posture see Table 6.1.

Irritability

Most babies cry at some time, but they are generally consolable either by picking them up and comforting them, changing their nappy or by feeding them. A baby who cannot be consoled may have an underlying reason for this (see Table 6.1).

Sleepy

Most babies sleep for most of the day, but they do tend to wake for feeds. Excessive sleepiness is abnormal. For causes see Table 6.1.

Inability to feed or suck

This may alert the practitioner to examine for prematurity (assess gestational age) and exclude physical anomalies such as cleft palate. Jaundice may also render the baby reluctant to feed, or there may be a neurodevelopmental abnormality requiring further investigation (Table 6.1).

Vomiting

Most babies will vomit at some time. Frequent large vomits are abnormal and a cause should be sought (Table 6.1).

Bile-stained vomit (green or yellow) is abnormal and is likely to indicate an intestinal obstruction.

Blood-stained vomit may be the result of ingestion of maternal blood, trauma or a coagulation problem (excluded by checking the clotting and the platelet count).

Abnormal movement

Asymmetry

Babies should be capable of moving both sides of their body to the same degree – not necessarily at the same time! If movement appears to be asymmetrical there may be an underlying cause (see Table 6.1).

Fits

At some point in time most babies will exhibit jerking movements. Determining which of these movements are normal and which are abnormal can be difficult. Jerking movements of the limbs that settle when the limb is held are usually not significant, but those that do not settle may well represent a fit. Other movements that may represent a fit include 'cycling' movements of the arms and legs. Sometimes the only evidence of a fit is a dusky (slightly cyanosed) baby, resulting from a brief cessation of breathing (an apnoea attack) caused by the fit. For causes of fits see Table 6.1.

Treat the fits if they are prolonged or are causing neonatal compromise (apnoea, cyanosis and distress).

Jittery

A 'jitter' is a rhythmical movement of the arms and legs that settles when the limbs are steadied. It can be a normal finding (an exaggerated normal response), but it may have an underlying cause (see Table 6.1).

Scalp

Bruises/swelling

Bruising and swelling are common responses to trauma. Both will resolve with time. Bruising may contribute to the development of jaundice.

Caput succedaneum (Figure 6.1)

This is subcutaneous oedema resulting from prolonged labour. It may present with or without bruising, and crosses suture lines. This is a benign finding that will resolve fairly quickly.

Cephalhaematoma (Figure 6.2)

Trauma causes subperiosteal haemorrhage confined to the skull bone(s). Swelling is contained within the suture lines but may be unilateral or bilateral. This is a benign finding that will gradually resolve and may contribute to the development of jaundice. The swelling should not increase in size after the delivery.

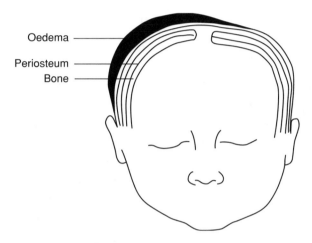

FIGURE 6.1 Caput succedaneum

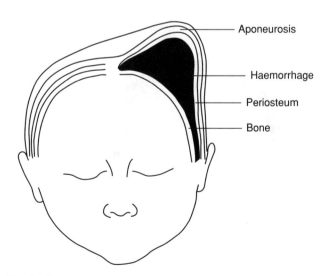

FIGURE 6.2 Cephalhaematoma

Subaponeurotic haemorrhage (Figure 6.3)

Trauma to the scalp causes a subaponeurotic haemorrhage not confined to a bone. The haemorrhage may be sufficient to necessitate resuscitation with intravenous fluids. Haemoglobin estimation may give some estimate of volume of blood loss, although the result may be misleading. Transfusion is likely to be necessary. A clotting screen may be abnormal owing to the consumption of clotting factors, and treatment with cryoprecipitate, platelets and vitamin K may be necessary.

Meningoceles and encephaloceles

These are usually found at the occiput in the midline. They are usually associated with a bony defect of the cranium. A meningocele contains meninges, i.e. the layers covering the spinal column, but does not contain any neural tissue. An encephalocele contains meninges and neural tissue. They may also be associated with an abnormal neurological examination. A cranial ultrasound will confirm the diagnosis, although a skull radiograph and cranial computerised tomography (CT) scan may also be required. Discussion and/or referral to a neurosurgeon will be necessary.

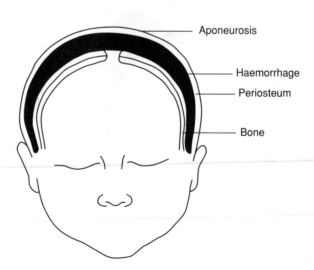

Aponeurosis

Haemorrhage

Periosteum

Bone

FIGURE 6.3 Subaponeurotic haemorrhage

Face

Asymmetry

May be the result of the baby lying awkwardly *in utero*, but it can occur with syndromes such as Goldenhar's syndrome (see p. 163), and it can occur in association with hemihypertrophy (enlargement of one side of the body). Hemihypertrophy may also be associated with nephroblastoma (a renal tumour).

In the case of a postural deformity, the only action necessary is to explain to the parents that this is usually a benign finding that will resolve fairly quickly. If there is associated hemihypertrophy a renal ultrasound scan should be arranged. It may be necessary to enlist the services of a geneticist to identify a syndrome if one is suspected. Severe facial abnormalities may benefit from referral to a craniofacial surgical team.

Small jaw

May be familial or it may occur as part of a syndrome, e.g. Pierre–Robin (see p. 160) syndrome. The first thing to do is to take a close look at the parents. If you suspect Pierre–Robin syndrome is likely, be sure to look for an associated cleft palate.

Dysmorphic facies

These may be familial, so always look at the parents. They can also occur in certain syndromes, e.g. Goldenhar's, Down's, Turner's (see p. 163), and in association with metabolic conditions, e.g. mucopolysaccharidoses and congenital hypothyroidism.

If you suspect a syndrome look for other features associated with the syndrome. Chromosome analysis may assist in confirmation or identification of a syndrome. It may be necessary to enlist the services of a geneticist to identify a syndrome if one is suspected.

Birthmarks (see Skin, p. 126)

There are many types of birthmarks, but those occurring most commonly in the neonatal period include the following:

Salmon patch naevus

Salmon patch naevus does not require intervention.

Port wine stain

Port wine stain in the distribution of the first branch of the trigeminal (third cranial) nerve may be associated with vascular malformation of the meninges and cerebral cortex on the same side. Radiological investigation, e.g. cerebral ultrasound, CT scan or magnetic resonance imaging (MRI), will help to exclude such involvement and should be considered. Referral to a dermatologist for cosmetic treatment should also be considered.

Strawberry haemangioma

This may need to be referred to a dermatologist if it involves the eyelid or has the potential to obstruct vision in the early years. Otherwise, after its rapid growth spurt, it should resolve.

Cavernous haemangioma

This should be referred to a dermatologist.

Nose

Obstruction

Failure of the nasal passages to become patent may cause obstruction (unilateral or bilateral choanal atresia) as may deviation of the nasal septum.

BILATERAL CHOANAL ATRESIA

Bilateral choanal atresia requires urgent treatment, which consists of establishing a patent airway and urgent referral to an ENT surgeon.

UNILATERAL CHOANAL ATRESIA

Unilateral choanal atresia requires referral to an ENT surgeon, but the urgency is not quite so great as with a bilateral atresia. A deviated nasal septum may require referral to an ENT surgeon.

Mouth

Neonatal teeth

Teeth present at or shortly after delivery are not common but should be referred to the orthodontic team, for they may be quite loose and can be inhaled if not removed electively.

Cleft lip

This condition is sometimes detected in the antenatal period, especially in maternity units where detailed anomaly ultrasound scans are routine. In such cases the baby would be automatically referred to and examined by a paediatrician. However, it is worth noting that women who have had scans during which the condition was not detected may feel confused and betrayed and will require a lot of support. Practitioners should be familiar with local policies and resources regarding

1 the timing of surgical closure of the cleft;
2 equipment to help with feeding difficulties;
3 photographs showing babies before and after surgical repair; and
4 local and national support groups (see Appendix 1).

Cleft lip can be familial, but it may occur as a result of chromosomal abnormalities, e.g. Patau's syndrome (see p. 161), or antenatal maternal medication, e.g. phenytoin.

Look carefully for an associated cleft palate and for other features that might suggest a syndrome. Early referral to a plastic surgeon is required in order that the optimal time for treatment can be discussed.

Cleft palate

Fifty per cent of cases involve both lip and palate. Cleft palate is associated with the same aetiology as cleft lip described above. Urgent referral to the 'cleft lip team' (plastic surgeon, ENT surgeon, audiologist, orthodontic surgeon, and speech therapist) should be made.

Cysts

Ranulae

Are mucus retention cysts and appear as blue lumps beneath the anterior part of the tongue. They may be large enough to displace the tongue posteriorly and interfere with respirations. In the event of this happening, they can be aspirated, but they are usually left alone if they do not interfere with feeding or breathing.

Ebstein's pearl

See Milia (p. 127).

Tongue

Cysts and dimples

During development the thyroid develops from an area along the tongue and migrates down the thyroglossal tract in the neck to its final position. Remnants of the thyroglossal tract can present as cysts and dimples. If a cyst is sufficiently large to cause problems with feeding or respiration, consideration should be made whether or not the cyst contains thyroid tissue before it is removed.

Tongue-tie

Is a term used to describe a condition in which the frenulum of the tongue is attached too far forward. It does not usually interfere with either speech or feeding and intervention is not usually recommended, as division of the frenulum is often associated with considerable haemorrhage.

Ears

Absence

This is a rare finding, and any baby with this defect should be referred to the ENT surgeon, plastic surgeon and the audiologist.

Abnormal shape

Dysmorphic ears can occur as a result of a syndrome, e.g. Treacher–Collins (see p. 159), may be developmental or may be familial. Any baby with such an abnormality should be referred to the ENT surgeon, plastic surgeon and the audiologist.

Position

Low-set ears may be indicative of a syndrome, e.g. Edward's syndrome.

Pre-auricular skin tags

Pre-auricular skin tags are not uncommon and are not always associated with abnormal hearing. If there are multiple skin tags, it is usually worthwhile requesting an audiology screen. All pre-auricular skin tags are best referred to the plastic surgeons for removal.

Pre-auricular dimples

Pre-auricular dimples are more likely to be associated with abnormalities of hearing, and any baby with this defect should be referred to the plastic surgeon and the audiologist.

Eyes

Discharge

Causes include infection (conjunctivitis) and blockage of the lachrymal duct. Despite the common nature of this symptom in neonates, it should be carefully monitored and appropriately investigated. If an infection is suspected because the discharge is profuse or purulent, the eye should be swabbed for bacterial and chlamydial infection and the baby should be started on topical antibiotics. Ointments are more effective in the treatment of eye infections as they remain in contact with the eye for a greater period of time. Infection can be gonococcal, staphylococcal or chlamydial.

Gonococcal infection usually manifests 2–5 days after delivery; the discharge is copious and purulent and occurs in association with oedema of the eyelids and conjunctiva. Intensive treatment of both eyes is necessary as the condition may lead to ulceration and perforation of the eye.

Staphylococcal conjunctivitis manifests 3–5 days after delivery and is less severe than gonococcal infection.

Chlamydial conjunctivitis usually occurs later than gonococcal and staphylococcal conjunctivitis. Isolation of the organism requires a conjunctival scrape sample to be analysed for intracellular inclusions. It will respond to erythromycin, but untreated it can cause damage to the eye. A blocked lachrymal duct usually becomes patent with time and rarely requires ophthalmic intervention to unblock it.

Confirmation of gonococcal or chlamydial infection in the neonate should be followed by counselling for the mother and her partner.

Ptosis

This is the term used to describe a drooping eyelid. It may be congenital. If the drooping lid covers the pupil, referral to an ophthalmologist is necessary in order that vision can be accurately assessed.

Squint

This is common in babies, but it is usually a transient finding which corrects itself within minutes. Epicanthic folds (see p. 72) and a broad nasal bridge can often produce an apparent squint. Few genuine squints are detected in the neonatal period, but if the practitioner is convinced that there is a persistent squint the baby is best referred to an ophthalmologist for an opinion.

Epicanthic folds

These are vertical pleats of skin that overlap the medial angle of the eye (see Figure 5.2). They are common in infants and may result in the illusion that there is a squint. They are a normal feature in the Mongoloid races and in Down's syndrome (see p. 157).

Anophthalmia

Absence of an eye can occur spontaneously or as part of a syndrome. It is usually associated with a shallow orbit, so for cosmetic reasons, and for examination of the normal eye, the baby should be referred to an ophthalmologist.

Microphthalmia

A small eye may occur as a result of congenital infection, e.g. rubella. It will almost certainly interfere with vision, so the baby should be referred to an ophthalmologist. It may be worth screening for evidence of congenital infection, and other features suggestive of congenital infection should be sought.

Macrophthalmia

A large eye most commonly occurs as a result of congenital glaucoma, a condition in which the drainage of fluid from the eye is obstructed so causing a build-up of pressure in the eye. The cornea may also appear hazy in association with congenital glaucoma. Referral to an ophthalmologist should be made as a matter of urgency.

Coloboma

Coloboma of the iris appears as a sector-shaped gap. That gap may extend posteriorly to include the ciliary body and choroid. It may be isolated or part of a syndrome. Referral to an ophthalmologist is necessary.

Aniridia

Absence of the iris can occur spontaneously or in association with nephroblastoma. Referral to an ophthalmologist is necessary and the kidneys should be scanned.

Heterochromia

An iris that has different pigment may not be apparent at birth but may develop as the eyes change from their newborn blue to their 'adult' colour.

Translucent iris

This occurs when there is reduced pigmentation of the iris, as occurs in albinism. Referral to an ophthalmologist is necessary.

White reflex (see Red reflex, p. 72)

> A white, rather than red reflex occurs with retinoblastoma (a retinal tumour) or scarring of the retina. The baby should be referred to an ophthalmologist for an opinion.

Cataract

> A cataract is an opacity of the lens. Cataracts vary in size and may be small dot-like lesions that cause no interference with vision, or they may be severe enough to produce a completely opaque lens. Some are hereditary; others are attributable to congenital infection, e.g. rubella, or biochemical imbalance, e.g. hypocalcaemia. The baby should be referred to an ophthalmologist to assess vision.

Neck

> The neck may be shortened in association with vertebral anomalies, e.g. Klippel–Feil syndrome. Turner's syndrome is associated with webbing of the neck. Damage to the sternomastoid muscle results in a sternomastoid tumour, a benign swelling within the muscle, and congenital torticollis ('wry neck').
>
> Abnormal swelling of the neck may result from a sternomastoid tumour or a cystic hygroma (a multicystic lesion of lymphatic origin). Branchial cleft remnants may present as dimples.

Limbs, including hands and feet

Absence and deformity

> Absence of a limb, hand or foot can result as part of a syndrome or may be an isolated abnormality that has occurred as a result of either a disruption in the sequence of development or an ischaemic event. Deformity can result from those same causes or as a result of intrauterine position.
>
> Deformity resulting from congenital absence of the fibula or radius can be associated with other abnormalities, e.g. low platelet count (thrombocytopenia). It can also result from congenital contractures (arthrogryposis). It should be noted that for all cases of limb deformities, other than those that are postural, early referral to an orthopaedic surgeon is essential.

Hands

Non-pitting oedema (lymphoedema) of the hands and feet is associated with both Turner's and Noonan's syndromes (see p. 158). The baby should be examined carefully for other features associated with the syndromes, and blood should be collected for chromosome analysis. The lymphoedema should settle with time.

Palmar creases

Single palmar creases are associated with Down's syndrome (see p. 157), but beware because 10% of the normal population have a unilateral single palmar crease and 5% have bilateral single palmar creases.

Feet

The feet may be abnormally positioned. Talipes equinovarus describes feet which are plantarflexed (turned downwards and inwards), whereas talipes calcaneovalgus describes feet which are dorsiflexed (turned upwards and outwards).

Digits

Polydactyly

Extra digits can occur spontaneously, as a familial trait or as part of a syndrome. Enquire whether polydactyly is a familial trait; if not, examine the baby carefully for other abnormal features. Bilateral polydactyly is often associated with renal anomalies, so arrange a renal ultrasound scan to exclude these.

A radiograph of the hand will reveal whether the extra digit has a bony component. If the extra digit has a bony component, refer the baby to an orthopaedic surgeon. Otherwise the anomaly can be referred to a plastic surgeon.

Syndactyly

Fusion of digits can occur spontaneously, as a familial trait or as part of a syndrome. Enquire whether syndactyly is a familial trait; if not, examine the baby carefully for other abnormal features.

A radiograph of the hand will reveal whether the syndactyly has fusion of the bones within. If there is fusion refer the baby to an orthopaedic surgeon. Otherwise the anomaly can be referred to a plastic surgeon.

Clinodactyly

Short inward curved little fingers can occur spontaneously, as a familial trait or as part of a syndrome, e.g. Down's syndrome. Enquire whether clinodactyly is a familial trait; if not, examine the baby carefully for other abnormal features. If this is the only finding, no action is necessary.

Skin

The skin may be affected by trauma, retention of secretions, hormonal instability, developmental abnormalities, congenital conditions and infection. Some of these produce similar findings, so they are grouped together by their appearances rather than their causes. Before these skin conditions can be described it is necessary to understand the associated terminology (Table 6.3).

Cuts and abrasions

These should be carefully observed as they serve as portals for infection. Discovery of any injuries found should always be carefully documented to avoid the potential for future dispute regarding their origin. (e.g. iatrogenic or possible non-accidental injury)

Bruises

Bruises may result from a difficult delivery or clinical interventions, e.g. taking blood. Most bruises are not sufficiently large to produce major problems, but as they are broken down they contribute to the bilirubin load and so to jaundice.

Petechiae

These are often evident following a precipitate delivery or if the umbilical cord was tight around the neck; they are usually on the face. However, they can also occur with thrombocytopenia and may be found in association with congenital infection, e.g. toxoplasmosis, rubella, cytomegalovirus, meningitis or herpes. Each of these congenital infections is associated with other abnormalities, which should be considered if the diagnosis is suspected.

TABLE 6.3 The skin: glossary of terms

Term	Meaning
Erythema	Superficial reddening of the skin
Petechiae	Fine purple/red non-blanching spots
Papula	Pimple, spot, small eruption on the skin
Vesicle	Blister, fluid-filled bubble on the skin
Pustule	Pimple containing pus
Macule	Dark blemish on the skin
Naevus	Birth mark comprising raised red area on the skin

Milia (papules)

These are small papules, white or yellow in colour, which usually appear grouped together. They are commonly found on the face, but can occur on the body. They are caused by the retention of sebaceous gland secretions when tiny follicular ducts become plugged. An Ebstein's pearl is a milia either on the hard palate of the mouth or on the penis. They usually resolve spontaneously within the first 8 weeks of life.

Miliaria

These are small vesicles with surrounding erythema which disappear when the skin cools. They are caused by blockage of sweat ducts with subsequent leakage into the epidermis.

Neonatal acne

This condition is characterised by small pustules with erythematous bases. It is caused by increased sebaceous gland activity secondary to maternal androgens and resolves with time.

Erythema toxicum neonatorum

This can occur anywhere on the body very shortly after birth and is characterised by pustules on erythematous macules. They can be fleeting and at times can appear quite angry looking, but the baby remains well at all times. They usually disappear within 2 weeks of birth.

Neonatal impetigo

Vesicles or pustules appear on an erythematous base and denude and begin to crust. It is caused by staphylococcal or streptococcal infection, and the baby is usually unwell. It is serious and highly infectious and requires treatment with intravenous antibiotics.

Congenital herpes

A vesicular eruption appears with surrounding erythema. There is usually multisystem involvement and there is a high morbidity and mortality rate. Rapid diagnosis and treatment is necessary if further progression is to be prevented. Treatment is with intravenous acyclovir.

Incontinentia pigmenti

Inflammatory vesicles develop within the first 2 weeks of life. These subsequently progress through several stages, including diffuse wart-like lesions, whorled hyperpigmentation and finally hypopigmentation in later childhood. It is found almost exclusively in girls.

Sucking blister

This is a blister without any surrounding inflammation and is the result of the fetus sucking the skin *in utero*. It resolves without treatment.

Epidermolysis bullosa

This is a group of blistering diseases differentiated from one another by histological criteria, mode of inheritance and healing capability. Blisters occur in response to varying degrees of contact and leave scarring. It is an inherited condition resulting in excessive response to trauma. Some types are associated with a high mortality because of complications and therefore suspected cases should be urgently referred to a specialist centre. Meticulous skin care and urgent treatment of skin infections may reduce the degree of scarring.

Lymphangioma circumscriptum

This collection of small vesicles occurs as a result of an abnormal collection of lymphatic channels that penetrate into subcutaneous tissues. No intervention is possible as surgery may be too difficult.

Neonatal Candida

This yeast infection occurs on the skin, causing redness (often with satellite lesions) and in the mouth, forming a white coating, which is not easily removed by scraping. It is caused by *Candida albicans* and left untreated it can result in poor feeding or a persistent nappy rash. Treatment with topical anti-fungals should eradicate the fungus, but precautions should be taken to prevent reinfection, e.g. the breast feeding mother must be treated, and teats and dummies should be cleaned thoroughly.

Hypopigmentation

ALBINISM

There is reduced pigmentation of skin, hair and/or retinae. It is a genetic condition. Referral to dermatologist (and ophthalmologist if there is eye involvement) is necessary.

ASH LEAF MACULES

These are hypopigmented areas of skin with an irregular outline, best seen with a Wood's (ultraviolet) lamp. They are characteristic of a neuro-cutaneous syndrome called tuberous sclerosis. The condition is associated with intracardiac lesions, abnormal cranial CT scan, a tendency to epilepsy and other skin abnormalities such as shagreen (sharkskin) patches.

Pigmentation

MONGOLIAN BLUE SPOTS

These are areas of blue-grey pigmentation, commonly found in infants of non-Caucasian parents. They are usually found over the back or buttocks, tending to fade during the first year of life, and are of no clinical significance.

CONGENITAL PIGMENTED NAEVI

These appear as pigmented plaques or papules of variable size and colour. The depth of tissue involvement may vary considerably. There is a risk of malignancy with time. The baby should be referred to a dermatologist.

CAFÉ AU LAIT SPOTS

These appear as light-brown coffee-like stains on the skin. More than six *café au lait* spots measuring greater than 1.5 cm suggests a diagnosis of neurofibromatosis. They are also associated with other conditions, namely tuberous sclerosis and Albright syndrome (a condition in which there can also be fibrous dysplasia of bone, precocious puberty and facial asymmetry).

SEBACEOUS NAEVUS OF JADASSOHN

This has the appearance of a collection of cholesterol deposits. It is yellow-brown or orange-pink and more commonly appears on the scalp or face. It may become malignant at puberty, and hence the baby should be referred to a dermatologist.

Vascular lesions

SALMON PATCH NAEVUS

This is a faint pink patch usually found on the nape of the neck, glabella or upper eyelid. Those on the nape of the neck persist, whereas the others usually disappear.

PORT WINE STAIN

This is a blue-purple, red or pink vascular marking that may darken with age. It can occur anywhere on the body. It may be associated with certain syndromes such as Edward's, Beckwith–Wiedemann and Sturge–Weber (port wine stain of the first branch of the trigeminal nerve with vascular malformations of the meninges and cerebral cortex on the same side).

STRAWBERRY HAEMANGIOMA

At birth this appears as a pale area with spidery blood vessels (telangiectasia). During the first 6 months it develops into a bright-red strawberry-like growth. It will subsequently involute. It results from an abnormal collection of capillaries and venules. It may obstruct vision or break down and become infected.

CAVERNOUS HAEMANGIOMA

This appears as a blue discoloration of the skin. It is an abnormal collection of larger vascular elements in the skin. It usually grows with the child. It may haemorrhage or cause high output cardiac failure and thrombocytopenia.

Ichthyosis

Ichthyosis is thickened, scaly, fish-like skin. It is inherited as a genetic condition. Topical agents may produce some symptomatic relief. Referral to a dermatologist may be needed.

Aplasia cutis

This condition is absence of the skin. It may be ischaemic in origin. It is associated with some syndromes. It usually heals spontaneously, although larger defects may require grafting.

Chest

Shape

UNDERDEVELOPED CHEST

A poorly developed chest wall may be the result of certain syndromes, e.g. Poland's syndrome or thoracic dystrophy (see p. 164).

HYPERINFLATION

The chest appears barrel shaped. It may occur as a result of a diaphragmatic hernia (a defect in the diaphragm allowing abdominal contents to pass into the chest) or air trapping, as occurs in meconium aspiration syndrome.

ASYMMETRY

The normal chest wall is usually symmetrical. For causes of asymmetry see Table 6.1.

Nipples

WIDELY SPACED NIPPLES

These are associated with chromosomal abnormalities, e.g. Turner's syndrome (see p. 158). It is wise to check the number of chromosomes if other features suggest a syndrome.

ADDITIONAL NIPPLES

Any associated breast tissue has as much of a risk of developing carcinoma than has normally positioned breast tissue. It may therefore be wise to refer to a surgeon for removal.

Cardiovascular system

Colour (see Observations, p. 65)

Heart rate and rhythm

The rate may be reduced with heart block, maternal medication or maternal systemic lupus erythematosus. It may be increased with thyrotoxicosis, maternal medication and supraventricular tachycardia (SVT).

Femoral pulses/pulse volume

Femoral pulse volume may be reduced or absent with left ventricular outflow obstruction, e.g. coarctation of the aorta, and poor left ventricular function, e.g. hypoplastic left heart. The pulse volume may also be reduced with sepsis.

Apical impulse

The apical impulse is the impulse felt when the hand is laid over the apex of the heart. It is normally palpable in the fifth intercostal space in the midclavicular line. For causes of a displaced apical impulse see Table 6.1.

Heaves/thrills

Left sternal heave is evidence of right ventricular hypertrophy.
Upper left parasternal systolic thrill occurs with pulmonary stenosis.
Lower left parasternal systolic thrill occurs with a ventricular septal defect.

Heart sounds

FIRST HEART SOUND

This may be quieter with a complete atrioventricular septal defect as the valve components may not close efficiently.

SECOND HEART SOUND

The aortic component of the second heart sound may be louder with aortic coarctation. The pulmonary component of the second heart sound may be louder and may precede the aortic component with pulmonary hypertension.

This may be heard when left ventricular filling is increased, e.g. persistent ductus arteriosus and ventricular septal defect.

FOURTH HEART SOUND

This is audible at the apex with aortic stenosis or systemic hypertension. It is audible over the right ventricle with pulmonary stenosis or pulmonary hypertension.

Murmurs

An ejection systolic murmur is caused by flow through one of the outflow valves, i.e. pulmonary or aortic. It does not necessarily indicate stenosis of that valve as it can occur with the increased blood flow through the pulmonary valve that occurs with an atrial septal defect.

A pansystolic murmur represents escape of blood from a ventricle into an area of low pressure, as occurs with an incompetent atrioventricular (mitral or tricuspid) valve or a ventricular septal defect.

An early diastolic murmur represents incompetence of the outflow valves, i.e. aortic or pulmonary valves.

A mid-diastolic murmur represents turbulent blood flow through the atrioventricular valves (mitral or tricuspid), as occurs when they are stenosed.

A presystolic murmur may occur when turbulence of blood at one of the atrioventricular valves (mitral or tricuspid) results during atrial contraction.

Respiratory system

Colour (see Observations, p. 65)

Respiratory effort and rate

RECESSION

This is the term used to describe in-drawing of the chest wall below (subcostal) and between (intercostal) the ribs. It occurs as result of increased work of breathing. For causes, see Table 6.1.

This is more of a 'moaning' noise heard at the end of each expiration. It represents air being exhaled against a partially closed glottis in an effort to increase the pressure in the terminal airways and so keep them inflated. For causes, see Table 6.1.

Respiratory pattern

For causes of apnoea, tachypnoea and grunting, see Table 6.1.

Air entry

This is usually symmetrical, but because of the relatively close proximity of the larger airways to the chest wall, the breath sounds may sound bronchial in nature, i.e. like those heard over the larynx or over consolidated tissue. This, combined with the relatively small surface area of the neonate's chest, makes it more difficult to differentiate between normal tissue and consolidated tissue by auscultation alone. Added sounds, e.g. crackles (crepitations), wheeze (rhonchi) and stridor, are significant. For causes of unequal air entry and additional sounds see Table 6.1.

Abdomen

Colour

A red or dusky abdomen is not normal and may indicate an inflamed bowel. It may also indicate ascending infection from the umbilicus. The baby should be examined carefully, paying particular attention to the presence of temperature instability, vomiting, jaundice, abdominal discomfort and the passage of faeces. For causes of a discoloured abdomen see Table 6.1.

Shape

THE SCAPHOID ABDOMEN

An in-drawn or sunken abdomen is referred to as scaphoid. It can betray the presence of a diaphragmatic hernia (a defect in the diaphragm allowing abdominal contents to pass into the chest). The baby should be examined carefully, paying particular attention to whether there is any respiratory compromise. Under these circumstances urgent chest and abdominal radiographs should be requested to exclude this diagnosis.

The presence of a distended abdomen may indicate an underlying obstruction. Pay particular attention to whether there is any vomiting, jaundice, abdominal discomfort and whether the baby has passed meconium/faeces.

In the presence of these symptoms an urgent abdominal X-ray should be requested to exclude a diagnosis of obstruction. X-ray may not be confirmatory so the opinion of a paediatric surgeon may be required.

This condition is rare, but represents the result of lax abdominal muscles. It is often associated with congenital megaureter, renal anomalies and bilateral undescended testes in the male. Renal ultrasound will detect small dysplastic (abnormally developed) kidneys and congenital megaureter (big ureter). The opinion of a paediatric surgeon or nephrologist will be required.

Organomegaly (enlarged organ)

Hepatomegaly and splenomegaly

For potential causes see Table 6.1.

Enlarged kidney(s)

This condition usually occurs secondary to hydronephrosis (dilatation of the ureter by urine), but can occur as a result of abnormal development, e.g. cystic dysplastic (abnormally formed) kidney, or nephroblastoma (renal tumour).

An urgent ultrasound is needed, and further information may be obtained by performing a micturating cystourethrogram (MCUG). A paediatric surgical opinion may be necessary for marked hydronephrosis and is definitely required for nephroblastoma.

Enlarged bladder

This is most obvious when there is bladder outlet obstruction, e.g.

posterior urethral valves or a neuropathic bladder, i.e. one with a faulty nerve supply. Examine the baby carefully, paying particular attention to the urinary stream, spine and the neurological examination.

An urgent ultrasound is needed, and further information may be obtained by performing an MCUG. A paediatric surgical opinion will be necessary for posterior urethral valves and may be necessary for a neuropathic bladder.

Masses

Mass is the term used for a unidentified swelling. The site of any mass is often a good indicator of its source; however, confusion can arise when an organ develops elsewhere and its natural course of migration is disturbed. Masses most commonly palpated in the abdomen include:

- hydroureter
- obstructed bowel
- ovarian cysts
- horseshoe kidney.

Abdominal X-ray and ultrasound will provide valuable information about the mass, but contrast studies may also be required, as may the assistance of a paediatric surgeon.

Tenderness

This is difficult to assess in a baby, but where there is obvious discomfort associated with palpation, this usually indicates underlying pathology, e.g. ischaemia, obstruction, trauma, etc. Check the maternal notes for evidence a traumatic delivery. Examine the baby carefully looking for evidence of temperature instability, vomiting, jaundice, passage of faeces, and trauma.

An infection screen will be indicated in conjunction with radiological investigation, e.g. ultrasound and X-ray.

Groin swelling

A hernia is a swelling usually containing bowel. Most are found in the groin and are reducible, i.e. can be gently pushed back from where it came. If it is not reducible the baby will require urgent referral to the paediatric surgeon. A reducible hernia will require an outpatient referral to the paediatric surgeon.

Absent femoral pulses

See Chest, Table 6.1.

Male genitalia

Scrotum

APPEARANCE

A small scrotum with no rugae may because there have never been testes within it. Examine the baby carefully to detect ectopic or maldescended testes. Absence of both testicles should alert the practitioner to the fact that the baby's sex may be indeterminate. This will necessitate careful examination of the baby and chromosomal analysis (see Bilateral absence of the testes, p. 138).

BIFID

Occasionally, the scrotum develops as a bifid (split) structure; the baby should be examined carefully to confirm that there are testes present in each half of it and that the rest of the genitalia are normal.

SWELLING

A large scrotum may be the result of a hydrocele. A hydrocele is a swelling in the groin or scrotum containing fluid. It can be distinguished from a hernia by shining a bright light source directly onto the overlying skin – a hydrocele will transilluminate (glow). It will not usually require attention, unless it causes compression of the testicle. It usually resolves with time.

PIGMENTATION

Pigmentation of the scrotum is common in babies born to parents who are not white. For other causes see Table 6.1.

DISCOLORATION

Discoloration of the scrotum occurs with a neonatal torsion (twist) of the testis; the testicle is usually painful in this condition. Ultrasound may provide useful information, but referral to a paediatric surgeon maybe necessary to exclude the condition.

Testes

UNILATERAL UNDESCENDED TESTICLE

In the absence of one testicle, the groin on the side of the absent testicle should be carefully palpated as the testicle may not have completed its descent from the posterior abdominal wall. It is also prudent to palpate just below the groin as the testicle may have descended abnormally to that area (see below).

If a testicle is undescended it may yet complete its descent, so it is worthwhile notifying the general practitioner rather than arranging a formal surgical follow-up. It must be made clear to the parents that the testicle should be descended by the age of 1 year or surgical intervention will be necessary to locate the testicle in the scrotum.

MALDESCENDED TESTICLE

If a testicle has descended abnormally and come to lie in the femoral triangle (the area directly below the groin), it should be discussed with a paediatric surgeon.

BILATERAL ABSENCE OF THE TESTES

Absence of both testicles should alert the practitioner to the fact that the baby's sex may be indeterminate. This will necessitate careful examination of the baby and further investigations. These investigations will include ultrasound of the pelvis and abdomen to locate female reproductive organs and/or undescended testes and chromosome analysis. The baby should then be discussed with an endocrinologist and a paediatric surgeon in the light of the examination findings and results of the investigations.

Penis

SIZE

The size may vary considerably, but if the penis still appears to be small when compared with centile charts for stretched penile length, the baby should be examined carefully. It may be worth discussing the baby's examination with an endocrinologist.

SHAPE

In the condition known as chordee the penis is tethered to the scrotum on its underside. This results in the penis being curved. This can lead to problems with erection later in life. The baby should be referred to a paediatric surgeon for correction.

Hypospadias is a term used to describe an abnormal shape to the penis. It may be merely a hooded appearance to the foreskin or an abnormality of shape in association with an abnormally placed meatus. An isolated hooded foreskin requires no intervention, but if it is associated with a malpositioned meatus surgery will be required, and referral should be made to a paediatric surgeon. The parents should be discouraged from having the baby circumcised as the foreskin is used in the repair procedure. As there are often associated renal abnormalities, a renal ultrasound should be requested.

POOR URINARY STREAM

May be the result of a narrow meatus or posterior urethral valves. Examine the baby carefully, paying particular attention to the foreskin and its opening. If ballooning of the foreskin occurs during urination, the baby's condition should be discussed with a surgeon. An urgent renal ultrasound will not show posterior urethral valves, but it may show resultant obstruction; an MCUG is necessary to exclude the diagnosis of posterior urethral valves.

Female genitalia

Labia

APPEARANCE

Pigmentation of the labia is common in babies born to parents who are not white. For other causes see Table 6.1.

SIZE

If the labia are large, this may alert the practitioner to the fact that there could be testes within them. They may also appear large in small for dates and preterm babies.

MASSES

There may be palpable testes within what appear to be the labia. Ultrasound of the pelvis and abdomen will help to identify female reproductive organs, if present.

Vagina

TAGS

These are often found in this area. They do not usually cause any problems and most can be left, as they become relatively smaller with time.

BLEEDING

Pseudo-menstruation can occur as a result of withdrawal from maternal hormones. It usually begins within the first 48 hours of delivery and may persist for up to 6 days. At times it can be quite heavy, but there are never frank clots present, although there may be some mucus.

Clitoris

SIZE

This is usually not particularly large, but in more preterm or small for dates babies it can appear large. If there are concerns about its size the baby should be examined carefully to confirm gender, taking particular care to check for testes.

Urinary meatus

POSITION

This is placed between the clitoris and the vaginal orifice. If urine is seen to dribble from any other point then a diagnosis of ectopic urethra should be considered and the baby should be examined carefully and discussed with a paediatric surgeon.

MICTURITION AND STREAM

It is unusual in the female baby to have any obstruction to the passage of urine. They are certainly not prone to posterior urethral valves.

Anus

Patency

A clearly imperforate anus requires urgent referral to the paediatric surgical team. In some cases of imperforate anus the anus may seem to be perforate, but there may be an obstruction at a higher level than is evident on external examination. If this is suspected referral to a paediatric surgeon is necessary.

Position of the anus

An anteriorly placed anus is commonly associated with problems. If the anus appears to be anteriorly placed, but the baby is not having any difficulties passing meconium, then an outpatient referral to the paediatric surgical team may be all that is necessary.

Meconium leaking from sites other than the anus is indicative of a fistula. The presence of a fistula is an indication for urgent referral and investigation.

Delayed passage of meconium

Delay in the passage of meconium beyond 24 hours should alert the practitioner to the possibility of problems such as Hirschprung's disease or imperforate anus, but it may also be delayed if the baby passed meconium *in utero*. Check the notes for evidence of meconium-stained liquor. Examine the baby carefully, paying particular attention to feeding, vomiting and abdominal distension. If the baby has severe abdominal distension and vomiting within hours of delivery, meconium ileus should be suspected, a symptom present in 20% of neonates with cystic fibrosis (Hull and Johnston 1993).

If there is associated abdominal distension, an X-ray may reveal evidence of obstruction, but it may be necessary to refer the baby to a paediatric surgeon.

Hips

Positive Ortolani's/Barlow's manoeuvre

These results are suggestive of congenital dislocation of the hip, and the baby should therefore be referred to an orthopaedic surgeon.

Asymmetry

Asymmetry may reveal an underlying congenital dislocation of the hip. Examine the baby carefully, paying particular attention to the result of Ortolani's manoeuvre (see Chapter 5). Refer to an orthopaedic surgeon if Ortolani's manoeuvre is positive.

Reduced range of movement

This may be indicative of a congenitally dislocated hip. Pay particular attention to skin creases and the result of Ortolani's manoeuvre. Refer to an orthopaedic surgeon if Ortolani's manoeuvre is positive.

Spine

Deformity

This may be the result of a hemi-vertebra or abnormal growth of the spine. This can occur spontaneously or in association with various syndromes. Examine the baby carefully, paying particular attention to the neurological examination. Discuss the findings with an orthopaedic surgeon.

Overlying marks or defects (including sacral dimples)

Such marks may indicate an underlying abnormality, e.g. spina bifida may be associated with an overlying tuft of hair or a naevus. Examine the baby carefully. Pay particular attention to the neurological examination. A sacral dimple with a visible base is insignificant. However, if the base can not be visualised, consider X-ray and ultrasound examination of the affected area. Discuss the baby with a neurosurgeon if findings are positive.

Central nervous system

Abnormal behaviour (see Observations, p. 65)

Abnormal behaviour may include:

1 a high-pitched cry
2 a lethargic baby
3 an irritable baby
4 a jittery baby
5 hypo- and hypertonia
6 asymmetrical reflexes
7 an inability to suck or feed.

Evidence of any of the above may indicate a neurological problem. Cranial ultrasound examination may reveal an underlying abnormality. The baby may need to be discussed with a paediatric neurologist and investigated further. See Table 6.1 for further details.

Check list

When the examination is complete, the practitioner must make sure that all that is referred to in the checklist at the end of Chapter 5 has been completed.

Specific abnormalities

Cardiac

Cyanotic congenital heart disease

TRANSPOSITION OF THE GREAT ARTERIES (FIGURE 6.4)

The aorta normally arises from the left ventricle and the pulmonary artery from the right ventricle, but in this condition the aorta arises from the right ventricle and the pulmonary artery from the left ventricle. *In utero* this does not pose a problem because pulmonary blood flow is small and there is movement across the patent ductus arteriosus and the patent foramen ovale, but once the baby is delivered and these two channels close two parallel circulations develop through the heart rather than one continuous circulation. The baby becomes increasingly cyanosed and heart failure develops. There is usually no associated murmur, but the second heart sound may be noted to be louder than usual because of the close proximity of the aorta to the anterior chest wall.

A chest radiograph may show a slightly enlarged heart with a narrow pedicle in association with heart failure. An electrocardiogram (ECG) is usually not useful at this stage. A hyperoxic test (undertaken in a neonatal unit) will confirm the presence of a cyanotic condition, but a cardiac ultrasound scan will confirm the diagnosis.

The baby requires urgent treatment with prostaglandin to re-open the duct and must be referred to a cardiologist for balloon septostomy and subsequent corrective surgery.

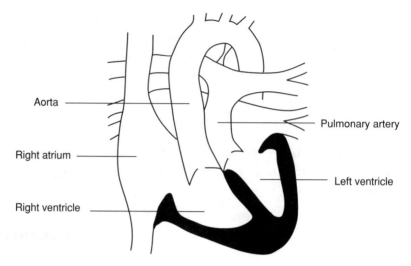

FIGURE 6.4 Transposition of the great arteries

TRICUSPID ATRESIA (FIGURE 6.5)

This condition results in cyanosis because of reduced blood flow to the lungs. Deoxygenated blood returning to the heart can only circulate by crossing through a patent foramen ovale. It then mixes in the left atrium with oxygenated blood from the lungs, and this mixture can only be circulated to the body via the aorta and to the pulmonary artery if there is a ventricular septal defect. There may not be a murmur, but there is only a single second heart sound.

A chest radiograph shows oligaemic lung fields and an ECG shows a superior axis and left axis deviation.

The baby requires urgent referral to a cardiologist for assessment.

PULMONARY ATRESIA (FIGURE 6.6)

This baby is dependent upon a patent ductus arteriosus to maintain pulmonary circulation. As the duct closes, the baby becomes increasingly cyanosed. There is usually no heart murmur, but there is only a single second heart sound.

A chest radiograph shows an enlarged right atrium in association with oligaemic lung fields. An ECG shows left ventricular hypertrophy.

The baby requires urgent treatment with prostaglandin and referral to a cardiologist for assessment.

FALLOT'S TETRALOGY (FIGURE 6.7)

This condition does not always present in the neonatal period. It consists of four abnormalities:

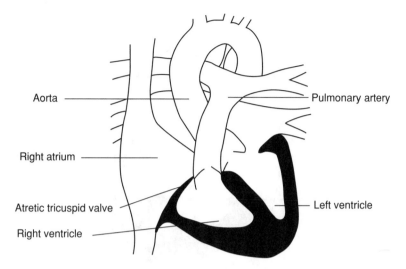

FIGURE 6.5 Tricuspid atresia

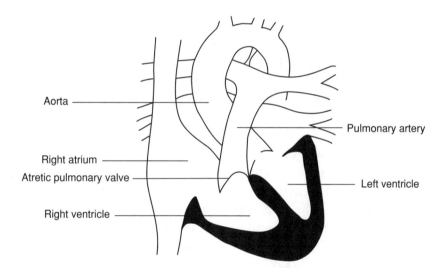

FIGURE 6.6 Pulmonary atresia

- a large ventricular septal defect
- an overriding aorta
- stenosis of the pulmonary valve or infundibulum
- a right ventricular hypertrophy.

The baby is usually pink, but with time develops cyanosis, which can become exacerbated owing to spasm of the pulmonary infundibulum. At this time a pulmonary stenosis murmur may be audible.

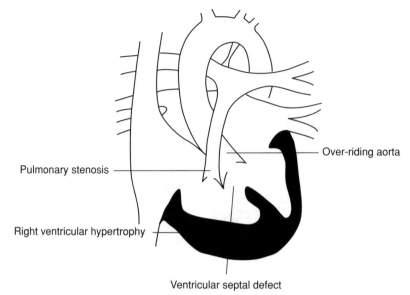

Pulmonary stenosis

Over-riding aorta

Right ventricular hypertrophy

Ventricular septal defect

FIGURE 6.7 Fallot's tetralogy

A chest radiograph shows a concave left heart border in association with oligaemic lung fields.

The baby requires urgent referral to the cardiologists. Treatment is usually surgical, but spasm may be prevented by the use of propranolol.

TOTAL ANOMALOUS PULMONARY VENOUS DRAINAGE (TAPVD)

This is a rare, but it can be mistaken for lung disease in a neonate. Abnormal drainage of the pulmonary veins to one of several places results in obstruction of the vessel(s) with subsequent pulmonary venous congestion. The baby is tachypnoeic and cyanosed. There may be a loud pulmonary second sound because of the pulmonary hypertension that develops as a result of the congestion.

Sometimes the chest X-ray is diagnostic, but the opinion of a cardiologist is usually required to confirm the diagnosis.

EBSTEIN'S ANOMALY

In this rare condition the baby may present with neonatal cyanosis. The right atrium is enlarged at the cost of the size of the right ventricle. The tricuspid valve is also abnormal and incompetent. The baby is cyanosed and there are additional heart sounds as well as the systolic murmur of tricuspid incompetence.

A chest radiograph shows a large globular ('wall-to-wall heart') with right atrial enlargement and oligaemic lung fields. An ECG shows tall P waves. The opinion of a cardiologist is usually required to confirm the diagnosis.

Acyanotic congenital heart disease

VENTRICULAR SEPTAL DEFECT (FIGURE 6.8)

This is the commonest of all congenital heart defects. It may be associated with other cardiac anomalies. It can occur in the membranous portion of the septum or in the muscular part. In the neonatal period these defects may be asymptomatic and there may not even be an audible murmur. In the larger defects, as the pulmonary vascular resistance falls, the flow across the defect (from left to right) increases, the lower left sternal pansystolic murmur develops and heart failure ensues.

A chest radiograph shows an enlarged heart and pulmonary plethora. A cardiac ultrasound scan will detect the defect.

The baby should be referred to a cardiologist for assessment; the urgency of referral depends on how well the baby is. Depending on the size and position of the defect, the baby may require urgent surgery, elective surgery or the defect may close spontaneously.

ATRIAL SEPTAL DEFECT (ASD) (FIGURE 6.9)

This defect is the result of failure of the atrial septum to develop correctly. The defect is low down and often involves the insertion of the mitral valve resulting in a cleft and incompetence. In addition to the murmur of the atrial septal defect, there is the apical pansystolic murmur of mitral incompetence.

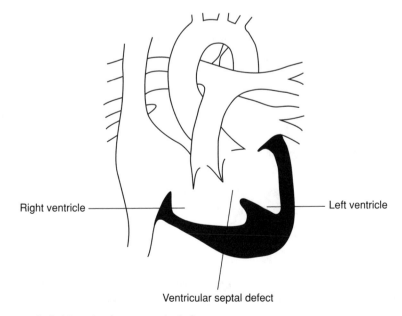

Right ventricle ————

Left ventricle

Ventricular septal defect

FIGURE 6.8 Ventricular septal defect

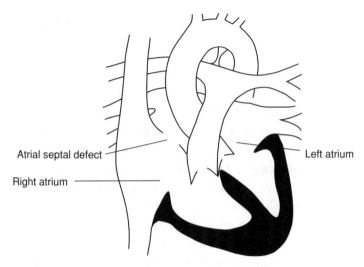

FIGURE 6.9 Atrial septal defect

A chest radiograph shows cardiomegaly and pulmonary plethora. An ECG shows left axis deviation and may show an RSR pattern in V_2 (anyone unfamiliar with ECGs should refer to a standard ECG textbook for further explanation).

The baby requires referral to a cardiologist for confirmation of the diagnosis and arrangements need to be made for early correction of the defect.

ATRIOVENTRICULAR CANAL DEFECT (FIGURE 6.10)

An extension of the ASD causing an ostium primum defect but involving the ventricular septum in addition to the atrial septum. The defect also involves both atrioventricular valves resulting in incompetence of both. The apical impulse is displaced as a result of cardiac enlargement. In the initial neonatal period, there may not be a murmur, but as pulmonary vascular resistance falls a murmur develops and the baby develops heart failure.

The chest radiograph shows marked cardiomegaly and pulmonary plethora, and the ECG has a superior axis.

The baby requires assessment by a cardiologist. Heart failure may be controlled by the use of diuretics, but a repair of the defect is required if complications are to be avoided.

PATENT DUCTUS ARTERIOSUS (FIGURE 6.11)

This is a relatively common heart lesion. It may present with heart failure in the neonatal period if the ductus is large. There is a wide pulse pressure; the apical impulse is displaced due to cardiac enlargement

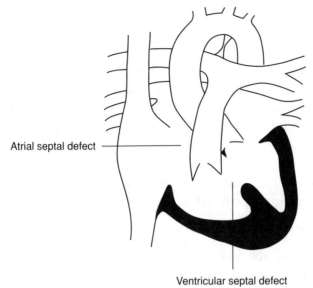

FIGURE 6.10 Atrioventricular canal defect

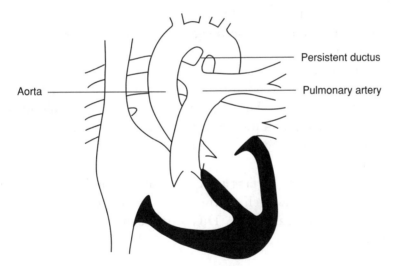

FIGURE 6.11 Patent ductus arteriosus

and there is a pulmonary systolic murmur. There may also be hepatomegaly and tachypnoea due to heart failure.

The chest radiograph shows cardiomegaly and pulmonary plethora. An ECG is often not helpful in the neonatal period.

Treatment with diuretics will control the heart failure and the duct may close in response to treatment with indomethacin, but it may be necessary to refer the baby for surgical ligation of the ductus.

Obstruction to outflow

PULMONARY STENOSIS

Narrowing of the pulmonary outflow tract can occur at different levels. Whatever the level, if the stenosis is severe it will present shortly after birth with cyanosis as a result of shunting across the foramen ovale and right-sided heart failure. There is usually a pulmonary systolic murmur audible and a right ventricular heave is palpable.

A chest radiograph may show an enlarged right atrium and right ventricle. An ECG shows right atrial and right ventricular hypertrophy. The baby requires referral to a cardiologist for assessment.

COARCTATION OF THE AORTA (FIGURE 6.12)

Narrowing of the descending aorta can occur at any point, but most commonly occurs close to the ductus arteriosus, distal to the left subclavian artery. Depending on the degree of coarctation, the baby may have few signs or may present in a collapsed state once the ductus closes. The one important thing in identifying a coarctation is the absence of femoral pulses, although these may be present while the ductus remains patent if the coarct is pre-ductal in position. There may be a murmur, which is best heard between the scapulae.

A chest radiograph is not usually of much use in the neonatal period and neither is an ECG, but a cardiac ultrasound scan should identify the lesion. A duct-dependent coarctation should respond to prostaglandin and requires urgent referral to a cardiologist for assessment.

Coarctation of the aorta is associated with Turner's syndrome, and other defects of the arch of the aorta are associated with other chromosomal anomalies, e.g. DiGeorge sequence with or without hypocalcaemia.

HYPOPLASTIC LEFT HEART

The diagnosis is sometimes made antenatally during ultrasound scanning. It is thought to result from an antenatal aortic outflow tract obstruction. This produces antenatal left ventricular hypertrophy, which subsequently results in a poorly functioning left ventricle postnatally. An unanticipated hypoplastic left heart presents as a baby with severe cardiac failure, i.e. tachypnoea, hepatomegaly, poor perfusion, etc.

A chest X-ray will show heart failure, but a cardiac ultrasound is diagnostic. The only thing that can help the baby is an urgent heart transplant, but a suitable donor is unlikely to be found.

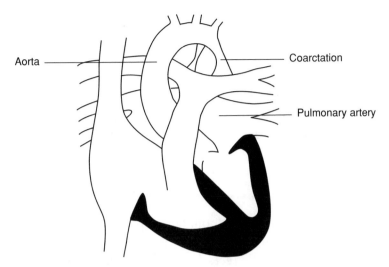

Aorta

Coarctation

Pulmonary artery

FIGURE 6.12 Coarctation of the aorta

Respiratory

Respiratory distress syndrome (RDS)

This condition is caused by reduced production of lung surfactant and occurs as a result of prematurity, hypoxia, acidosis or maternal diabetes. There is also a condition called congenital surfactant deficiency. Surfactant deficiency makes the lungs more difficult to expand and increases the work of breathing. The baby becomes cyanosed, has subcostal recession and tachypnoea, and may have an expiratory grunt.

A chest radiograph shows a classical ground glass appearance. Blood gas analysis will show a respiratory acidosis and hypoxia. This will become more marked and often requires treatment with respiratory support, artificial surfactant and intravenous fluids. As the condition is difficult to distinguish from congenital pneumonia it is usual for the baby to be commenced on intravenous benzylpenicillin.

The natural progression of the disease is for it to begin to resolve any time up to 72 hours of age, but it can be quite variable. In some babies the illness can be so severe that death is inevitable.

Congenital pneumonia

This infection is commonly associated with prolonged rupture of membranes. The responsible organism is not always isolated, but the organism most commonly causing pneumonia is the group B

Streptococcus. Other organisms include *Escherichia coli*, *Listeria monocytogenes* and staphylococci. As with respiratory distress syndrome, the baby is cyanosed with tachypnoea and recession. There may also be an expiratory grunt.

A chest radiograph will show the pneumonia and an arterial blood gas may show hypoxia and respiratory acidosis. The baby requires treatment with antibiotics and may require intravenous fluids and respiratory support.

Pneumothorax

A pneumothorax is not uncommon, but, depending on the size of the pneumothorax, the symptoms may vary in severity. The baby is usually tachypnoeic. There may be recession, cyanosis, grunting and unequal air entry. If the pneumothorax is sufficiently large, the chest will transilluminate with a cold light source.

A baby who is relatively well but has respiratory symptoms can be X-rayed, and the findings will be characteristic. In a baby who has collapsed as a result of a pneumothorax, there will not be sufficient time to arrange a chest radiograph, but its presence can be confirmed by transillumination and immediate action can be taken. A small pneumothorax will resolve spontaneously, but a larger symptomatic one will require treatment.

Choanal atresia

This may be bilateral or unilateral. A bilateral atresia will present early on with cyanosis and even obstructive apnoea. A unilateral atresia may come to light at a later stage. Unilateral atresia can be confirmed by obstructing each nostril in turn. When the patent nostril is obstructed, the baby will behave as if it has a bilateral atresia.

Insertion of an oropharyngeal airway will alleviate the obstruction temporarily, but the baby will require urgent referral to an ENT surgeon. CT scan usually confirms the atresia.

Gastrointestinal

Oesophageal atresia (OA) and tracheo-oesophageal fistula (TOF)

There are many different combinations of abnormalities of the oesophagus and trachea, but the main one is a blind-ending upper oesophagus in association with a communication between the lower oesophagus and the trachea. The oesophageal atresia may be diagnosed antenatally by the presence of polyhydramnios. Postnatally, the diagnosis is often made following choking or cyanotic episodes as a result of the baby being unable to swallow his own secretions.

If the diagnosis is suspected, the first priority is to protect the airway by commencing frequent suction of the pharynx. The baby should be carefully examined to exclude other abnormalities (anal, cardiac, skeletal and genitourinary). The diagnosis can be aided by attempting to pass a wide-bore (FG 10 or 12) radio-opaque nasogastric tube. Inability to pass the tube into the stomach is strong evidence for the presence of atresia, although presence of a TOF with no OA may allow a nasogastric tube to be passed; therefore, diagnosis should be confirmed by X-ray. The presence of gas in the bowel, despite an atresia, is confirmation that there is a tracheo-oesophageal fistula.

The baby requires urgent referral to a paediatric surgeon for division of the fistula and repair of the atresia, which may be difficult if the two ends of the oesophagus are not close to each other. Other abnormalities should not be forgotten and should be dealt with appropriately.

Diaphragmatic hernia

This hernia may be diagnosed antenatally, but some may present at delivery as a difficult resuscitation or even later with tachypnoea. The majority are left sided and so are associated with displacement of the heart sounds and apical impulse to the right. There is also reduced air entry on the left and a scaphoid abdomen.

The baby should be resuscitated and then examined carefully for other abnormalities. A chest radiograph will confirm the diagnosis. Once confirmed, a large-bore nasogastric tube should be inserted into the stomach and allowed to drain freely to avoid accumulation of air and its passage into the hernia, which would compromise breathing further. There is often associated pulmonary hypoplasia and the baby may require ventilation.

The baby requires urgent referral to a paediatric surgeon who is experienced in dealing with the anomaly.

Duodenal atresia

This condition is a relatively high obstruction and as such its presence may not be recognised early on because it is less likely to cause marked abdominal distension and may not necessarily be associated with bile-stained vomiting. Any distension that occurs is restricted to the epigastrium, but may be associated with visible peristalsis.

The baby should be examined carefully as the abnormality is associated with Down's syndrome. An abdominal radiograph will show the classical 'double bubble' of duodenal atresia.

The baby requires urgent referral to a paediatric surgeon for further investigations and repair of the lesion.

Imperforate anus

Like oesophageal atresia, an imperforate anus is not always apparent, and there are numerous anatomical variations. The anomaly may be obvious when the baby is first examined, but it may only become apparent when the baby develops abdominal distension or fails to pass meconium. The 'high' imperforate anus is the least obvious and may or may not be associated with a recto-vaginal or recto-vesical fistula. The 'low' anomaly may merely consist of a membrane covering the anus.

The baby should be examined carefully as the anomaly may be part of a collection of abnormalities. An abdominal radiograph will show intestinal obstruction and the absence of gas in the rectum. He will require urgent referral to a paediatric surgeon for further investigation and treatment.

Gastroschisis

A defect in the anterior abdominal wall allows the bowel to protrude through it. Unlike exomphalos there is no sac covering the bowel and this abnormality is not usually associated with other abnormalities.

The defect allows major fluid and heat loss to occur, so the exposed bowel is best covered with clingfilm to minimise this, and intravenous access should be established. Urgent transfer to a paediatric surgical unit is necessary.

Exomphalos

Abdominal contents protrude through the abdominal ring into the umbilical cord. They are covered with a transparent sac. There is a risk of heat and fluid loss, so the contents are best covered with clingfilm and intravenous access should be gained. There is an association with chromosomal, cardiac, gastrointestinal and genitourinary abnormalities as well as with Beckwith–Wiedemannn syndrome.

The baby should be examined carefully to exclude other abnormalities and the blood sugar should be monitored to exclude hypoglycaemia. It may be necessary to take blood for chromosome analysis and to arrange further investigations to exclude associated abnormalities. The baby should be referred to a paediatric surgeon for repair of the defect.

Genitourinary

Posterior urethral valves

This is a condition that affects males and results in obstruction to the flow of urine with hydronephrosis. It is commonly suspected antenatally by the presence of hydronephrosis on antenatal ultrasound. It can cause impaired renal function, but this may be reversible with drainage and careful attention to fluid and electrolyte balance.

The condition is confirmed by micturating cystourethrogram (MCUG). The baby requires urgent referral to a paediatric surgeon for disruption of the valves.

Ambiguous genitalia

This condition can occur as a result of many different problems, e.g. chromosomal, hormonal, etc. Whatever the reason, it is important to the parents for the baby to be assigned to one or other gender as quickly as possible. However, the gender to which the baby is assigned requires careful consideration of three basic things:

1 genetic sex, i.e. chromosomal karyotype;
2 gonadal sex, i.e. the presence or absence of testes, which will only develop in response to the H–Y antigen; and
3 functional sex, i.e. the usefulness of the organs present.

Check the maternal notes for evidence of family history of ambiguous genitalia or neonatal death and exposure to drugs in pregnancy. Examine the baby carefully, paying particular attention to the appearance and size of the genitalia and other abnormalities.

Blood should be taken for chromosome analysis, urea and electrolytes, plasma ACTH (adrenocorticotrophic hormone) and

17-hydroxyprogesterone levels. A pelvic ultrasound will identify the female reproductive organs, if present. Other radiological investigations may be necessary. The baby should be discussed with an endocrinologist and a paediatric surgeon as a matter of urgency.

Hypospadias

The majority of these anomalies are glandular or coronal and merely require the practitioner to confirm that the baby is passing urine adequately. More severe forms may be associated with other abnormalities, e.g. renal, intersex, etc.

The baby should be examined carefully. If the hypospadias is more severe, a renal ultrasound should be arranged. The parents of a baby with hypospadias which is not glandular should be encouraged to avoid having their baby circumcised as the foreskin may be required to repair the abnormality. The baby should be referred to a paediatric surgeon for repair of the abnormality.

Epispadias

This condition affects more boys than girls. In the male with epispadias, the urethra is a strip of mucosa on the dorsum of the penis. In the female, there is a double clitoris and the urethra is split dorsally.

The baby should be examined carefully to exclude other abnormalities. A renal ultrasound should be requested, and the baby requires urgent referral to a paediatric surgeon.

Bladder extrophy

This condition affects boys more frequently than girls. There is complete epispadias, exposure of the bladder mucosa on the anterior abdominal wall and division of the symphysis pubis.

There may be other abnormalities, so careful examination should take place to exclude other abnormalities. A renal ultrasound should be requested, and the baby requires urgent referral to a paediatric surgeon.

Musculo-skeletal

Some babies with skeletal dysplasias may present difficulties at delivery requiring resuscitation. Pulmonary hypoplasia may result from external compression as a result of a small chest cage, as seen in the lethal condition thanatophoric dwarfism.

Achondroplasia

This is a dominantly inherited condition, but it may also occur as a result of a spontaneous mutation. There is a normal-size trunk in association with short limbs and a large head. There may be hydrocephalus.

If either parent has achondroplasia, then that is the likely diagnosis. Skeletal X-ray changes are characteristic and a cranial ultrasound will exclude hydrocephalus. Paediatric follow-up is necessary, although the outcome is usually good.

Osteogenesis imperfecta

This may result in multiple fractures of the long bones and ribs antenatally with subsequent deformities.

The abnormality may be diagnosed *in utero*, but postnatally the diagnosis can be confirmed by radiography of the bones. The baby requires referral to an orthopaedic surgeon.

Specific syndromes

The practitioner should ensure whenever a syndrome has been confirmed that parents are referred to a geneticist for counselling.

Down's syndrome

Down's syndrome results from additional genetic material from chromosome 21. The common form (94%) consists of the addition of a complete chromosome 21 to the chromosome complement, i.e. trisomy 21, but less common forms are the result of partial duplication of genetic material from chromosome 21. The incidence of Down's syndrome was 1 in 660 newborns (Jones 1997), but this will have been altered by the introduction of antenatal screening and selective termination of some fetuses. The majority of cases can be diagnosed clinically, but chromosome analysis allows confirmation of any less obvious cases. The clinical features most commonly found at birth include:

- craniofacial: flat facial profile, upward-slanting eyes
- eyes: inner epicanthic folds, Brushfield spots (speckling of the iris)
- neuromuscular: hypotonia
- hands and feet: relatively short metacarpals and phalanges, clinodactyly (inward curving) of the fifth finger, a wide gap between the first and second toes, single palmar crease and abnormal dermatoglyphics.

There may be an associated cardiac anomaly (most commonly complete atrio-ventricular septal defect or ventricular septal defect) and gastrointestinal anomaly (duodenal atresia or Hirschprung's disease).

Blood should be taken for chromosome analysis. An ECG may assist in excluding certain cardiac abnormalities, but referral to a paediatric cardiologist is advisable. The baby will require paediatric follow-up, as there will be developmental delay.

Turner's syndrome

Turner's syndrome is the result of the absence of a sex chromosome. The best known karyotype is XO, in which there is complete absence of a sex chromosome, but the syndrome can result from a partial deletion of a sex chromosome or from a mosaic genotype in which there is absence of sex chromosomes in some cells and not in others. The estimated incidence is 1 in 2000 live-born females (Jones 1997). The clinical features most commonly found at birth include:

- growth: small stature
- hands: lymphoedema, narrow hyperconvex nails
- skeletal: cubitus valgus
- thorax: widely separated nipples
- neck: webbing of the neck, low posterior hairline
- facies: relatively small mandible.

There may be an associated cardiac anomaly (most commonly bicuspid aortic valve and coarctation) and renal anomalies (horseshoe kidney) and there will be short stature and infertility.

Blood should be taken for chromosome analysis. A renal ultrasound scan will exclude horseshoe kidney. Referral to a paediatric cardiologist is advisable to exclude coarctation of the aorta. The baby will require paediatric follow-up as developmental delay is common and the input of a paediatric endocrinologist will also be required.

Noonan's syndrome

This consists of phenotypical features of Turner's syndrome in a male baby with cryptorchidism (bilaterally impalpable testes). It usually occurs sporadically, but apparent autosomal dominant inheritance has been documented and a gene for the disorder has been mapped. The clinical features most commonly found at birth include:

- skeletal: cubitus valgus
- thorax: shield chest and pectus excavatum or pectus carinatum
- neck: webbing of the neck, low posterior hairline
- facies: relatively small mandible, hypertelorism
- genitalia: small penis, cryptorchidism.

The most commonly associated cardiac abnormality is pulmonary valve stenosis. There is also an increased incidence of coagulation and platelet defects.

Blood should be taken for chromosome analysis and molecular genetics. Referral to a paediatric cardiologist is advisable. The baby will require paediatric follow-up.

Treacher–Collins syndrome (mandibulofacial dysostosis)

This is an autosomal dominant condition, although it can occur sporadically. In some of the cases there is an association with a particular gene mutation. The clinical features most commonly found at birth include:

- craniofacial: malar hypoplasia, mandibular hypoplasia, cleft palate, downward-slanting eyes
- ear: malformation of auricles
- eye: lower lid coloboma, absence of lower eyelashes.

The condition can be so severe that it causes problems with airway patency. There is often associated deafness.

In the first instance, the priority is to maintain the airway if there are any difficulties with this. Take a look at both parents – either may

159

have the condition. Blood should be taken for molecular genetics. The baby will require an audiology assessment, and it may be necessary to refer him to an ENT surgeon. Paediatric follow-up will be necessary.

Pierre–Robin syndrome

Pierre–Robin syndrome comprises:

- craniofacial: small jaw (micrognathia), a midline cleft palate and a protruding tongue (glossoptosis).

These features can occur to a greater or lesser degree. The main problem is that of airway obstruction secondary to the tongue falling back and obstructing the oropharynx. The baby can also experience problems with feeding.

This will require referral to an ENT surgeon, speech therapist and orthodontic surgeon. The small jaw may also require referral to a craniofacial team.

Apert's syndrome (acrocephalosyndactyly)

This is an autosomal dominant condition, but the majority of cases are sporadic. It is associated with a particular gene mutation. The clinical features most commonly found at birth include:

- craniofacial: short anteroposterior diameter, high forehead, flat occiput, craniosynostosis (premature fusion of suture) of the coronal suture, cleft palate, downward-slanting eyes.

Blood should be taken for molecular genetics. The premature fusion of sutures puts the growing brain at risk of compression, so it is necessary to refer the baby to a neurosurgeon for their opinion.

- hands and feet: syndactyly.

Syndactyly will require referral to an orthopaedic surgeon. The baby will also require paediatric follow-up, as mental deficiency is common.

Crouzon's syndrome (craniofacial dysostosis)

This is an autosomal dominant condition with variable expression, but it can occur sporadically. It is associated with a mutation of the same gene responsible for Apert's syndrome. The clinical features at birth include:

- craniofacial: ocular proptosis, hypoplasia of the maxilla, high forehead, craniosynostosis (coronal, lambdoid and sagittal)

Blood should be taken for molecular genetics. It will be necessary to refer the baby to a neurosurgeon for an opinion, as progressive intracranial hypertension will develop if the craniosynostosis is not treated. The baby will also require paediatric follow-up.

Patau's syndrome

Patau's syndrome occurs in 1 in 5000 births (Jones 1997). It results from trisomy for all or most of chromosome 13. The majority (82%) of these babies die within the first month of life. The clinical findings at birth include:

- craniofacial: microcephaly, narrow palpebral fissure, depressed saddle nose, high philtrum, cleft lip, cleft palate
- ears: low-set, abnormal helices
- eyes: microphthalmia, colobomata of iris
- hands and feet: flexion and overlapping of the fingers, polydactyly
- genitalia: cryptorchidism.

Cardiac abnormalities such as ventricular septal defect, patent ductus arteriosus and atrial septal defect are common. Incomplete development of the forebrain is also a common finding.

Examine the baby carefully. Blood should be taken for chromosome analysis. The baby will require referral to a paediatric cardiologist to exclude a cardiac anomaly. He will also require a cranial ultrasound scan and paediatric follow-up.

Edward's syndrome

Edward's syndrome had an incidence of 3 per 1000 newborn babies (Jones 1997), although with antenatal screening and selective termination this incidence will have been reduced. It results from trisomy for all or most of chromosome 18. The majority (90%) die within the first year of life. The clinical features found at birth include:

- growth: intrauterine growth retardation
- craniofacial: micrognathia, short palpebral fissure, epicanthic folds, narrow bifrontal diameter, prominent occiput
- ears: low-set
- hands: flexion deformity of the fingers
- feet: rocker bottom feet with dorsiflexed big toes
- genitalia: cryptorchidism.

Cardiac abnormalities are common and include ventricular septal defect, atrial septal defect and patent ductus arteriosus. Mental deficiency is common.

Examine the baby carefully. Blood should be taken for chromosome analysis. The baby will require referral to a paediatric cardiologist to exclude a cardiac anomaly. He will also require paediatric follow-up.

Cri du chat *syndrome*

This results from a partial deletion of chromosome 5. Approximately 85% result spontaneously. Clinical findings at birth include:

- growth: low birth weight
- craniofacial: microcephaly, hypertelorism, downward-slanting eyes, facial asymmetry
- ears: low set
- hands: single palmar crease, abnormal dermatoglyphics
- general: cat-like cry
- neuromuscular: hypotonia.

There also appears to be an increase in the incidence of congenital heart disease (variable abnormalities). All babies subsequently go on to develop learning difficulties.

Blood should be taken for chromosome analysis. Paediatric follow-up is essential.

Goldenhar's syndrome (hemifacial microsomia)

This results from abnormalities in the development of structures that are derived from the first and second branchial arches. Most cases occur sporadically, but there is a risk of recurrence in first degree relatives of about 2%. Clinical features evident at birth include:

- facial: hypoplasia of malar, maxillary or mandibular region, macrostomia.
- ear: microtia (small ear), pre-auricular tags or pits.

There are often associated abnormalities of the vertebrae (hemivertebrae) and abnormalities of the eye, such as microphthalmia or dermoids. There is also an increased incidence of cardiac abnormalities (ventricular septal defect, patent ductus arteriosus, Fallot's and coarctation), and renal anomalies (ectopic kidneys, reflux and dysplasia) are also common.

A renal ultrasound scan will exclude most of the associated renal anomalies. A paediatric cardiologist will detect cardiac anomalies. Cosmetic surgery will probably be necessary as will assessment of hearing. Paediatric follow-up should be arranged.

Möebius sequence (sixth and seventh nerve palsy)

This occurs as a result of one of four different problems:

1 hypoplasia or absence of the nerve nuclei in the brain;
2 destructive degeneration of the nerve nuclei in the brain;
3 peripheral nerve involvement;
4 myopathy.

It most commonly occurs sporadically, but in some cases it can be familial with an autosomal dominant inheritance. The clinical features at birth include:

- facial: expressionless facies (facial palsy), micrognathia.

Paediatric follow-up is required, as some cases have associated learning difficulties.

Poland's syndrome

In this condition the fullness of the upper part of the chest is lacking as a results of hypoplasia or absence of the pectoralis major muscle. There may be associated anomalies, e.g. hypoplasia/absence of the nipple and areola, distal limb hypoplasia (syndactyly/oligodactyly) and renal anomalies. A renal ultrasound should be requested.

Thoracic dystrophy

The chest appears elongated and thin. Respiratory compromise may be sufficient to cause respiratory distress and even death.

Beckwith–Wiedemann syndrome

Clinical findings at birth include:

- abdominal: exomphalos
- growth: the baby is usually large for dates
- metabolic: there are often problems with glucose metabolism
- ears: there is a characteristic skin crease on the lobe.

The baby's blood sugar should be monitored carefully and hypoglycaemia should be dealt with appropriately. A renal ultrasound should be performed as there is a risk of nephroblastoma. The baby will require paediatric follow-up.

DiGeorge sequence

Clinical findings at birth include:

- immunological: T-cell defects
- cardiac: aortic arch abnormalities, e.g. coarctation
- metabolic: hypoparathyroidism, leading to hypocalcaemia.

Calcium levels should be monitored closely and hypocalcaemia treated appropriately. As there is a risk of an aortic arch anomaly the baby should be referred for an urgent cardiac opinion. The baby will also require immunological investigations and paediatric follow-up.

Summary

We have explored the nature and initial management of some of the major abnormalities that may be suspected or discovered during the first examination of the newborn. Thankfully most babies are born perfectly healthy. However, the practitioner examining the baby must acknowledge that her care during this examination has the potential to make a valuable contribution to the future health and wellbeing of the neonate. The next chapter focuses on professional accountability and effective clinical practice in relation to the first examination of the newborn.

Chapter 7

Accountability and effective care

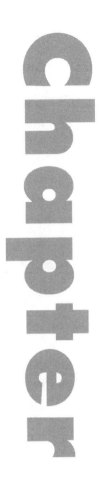

- Introduction
- Acknowledging professional responsibilities and boundaries
- Accountability
- Achieving and maintaining best practice
- Conclusion

Introduction

Although the purpose of the first examination of the newborn is to confirm normality, there are some potentially life-threatening conditions, such as some forms of congenital heart disease, which are not evident in the first 24 hours of the baby's life and therefore would not be detected (MacKeith 1995). Where the practitioner performing this clinical examination of the baby is new to the role, it is likely that she will have some concerns about the risk of litigation in the event of an abnormality being missed. For example:

> What is the legal position of a practitioner who does not detect a congenital condition in a baby during the first examination of the newborn?

It is therefore essential that this examination is performed with competence and an appreciation of the practitioner's accountability. Practitioners must recognise and acknowledge the responsibility that they carry (Michaelides 1997).

The aim of this chapter is, therefore, to acknowledge the role and responsibilities of practitioners who undertake the first examination of the newborn and to remind them of their professional, legal and employment accountability. The main focus of the second half of the chapter is to illustrate how the practitioner can take positive steps to increase the effectiveness of the first examination of the newborn, and it includes issues such as gaining and maintaining competence. It is important before these concepts are explored, that practitioners appreciate the role of the various members of the multidisciplinary team who have had responsibility for the first examination of the newborn.

Acknowledging professional responsibilities and boundaries

The role of the midwife encompasses physical examination and care of the newborn (UKCC 1998), and this skill is taught within the pre-registration midwifery programmes. This initial examination is undertaken shortly after the birth in order to confirm normality and identify readily apparent physical abnormality such as cleft lip or spina bifida. It does not, however, encompass the detailed examination of the heart, lungs, eyes, abdomen or hips that a paediatrician traditionally undertakes, usually within the first 24 hours, *the first examination of the newborn.*

In order for the registered nurse or midwife to undertake such an examination, a course of education, supervised practice and assessment of competence must be undertaken. Such an adjustment to the scope of professional practice, however, should only be undertaken if the following principles apply:

- patient care will be enhanced;
- existing care is not compromised;
- limits of practice are acknowledged;
- competence is maintained; and
- accountability for practice is borne.

Such expansion of professional practice should fulfil the framework outlined in the document *The Scope of Professional Practice* (UKCC 1992) and only be undertaken in the full knowledge and agreement of the hospital trust's legal department, as it is the trust who will assume vicarious liability if a parent sues for damages. It should be supported by a locally agreed policy and medical colleagues should ideally be involved in all preparations for adjustments to the scope of professional practice that potentially affect them. Nurses and midwives will continue to need their skill and expertise to support their daily practice, and every effort should be made to enhance the relationship rather than jeopardise it.

The fact that nurses and midwives have taken on some aspects of the doctor's role is not a new concept, for example the emergency nurse practitioner (Tye *et al.* 1988). Such extensions to the scope of professional practice help facilitate the provision of client-centred care through increasing the choices available for patients, provide more continuity of care and reduce the length of time that patients wait to be seen (McKenna *et al.* 1994).

We have explored issues relating to who undertakes the first examination of the newborn, and it is now appropriate that accountability within this role is further clarified.

Accountability

Accountability is defined in the 1993 *Oxford Dictionary* as 'answerability, responsibility, liability, culpability' and is an integral part of clinical practice. This section will consider the concept of accountability as it applies to the professional practice of doctors, nurses, midwives and health visitors. It is necessary to consider the three components to which professionals must conform:

1 professional accountability;
2 legal accountability; and
3 terms of employment.

Professional accountability

The regulatory body for nurses, midwives and health visitors is the United Kingdom Central Council (UKCC), and it defines the standards of conduct for these professions, exercising its powers conferred on it by the Nurses, Midwives and Health Visitors Act 1997. The General Medical Council (GMC) fulfils a similar remit for the medical profession.

The first examination of the newborn is not currently part of the role of *all* midwives or neonatal nurses. However, the midwife is an autonomous practitioner accountable for her practice within the bounds of normality. The activities of a midwife are defined in the European Union Midwives Directive 80/155/EEC Article 4 and outlined in the Midwives rules and code of practice (UKCC 1998). These activities include 'to examine and care for the newborn infant', and the directive provides a legal framework for practitioners to develop clinical skills in this aspect of their role. Where deviations from normal do occur, the practitioners must refer to an appropriate practitioner (UKCC 1998).

The Code of Professional Conduct for the Nurse, Midwife and Health Visitor (UKCC 1992: 1) states that 'as a registered nurse, midwife or health visitor, you are personally accountable for your practice ...' and clearly states how this should be exercised. Accountability applies to all aspects of practice in which the professional makes judgements and takes action as a result of those judgements, for example giving analgesia to a patient in pain. The professional is answerable for the actions taken and these should always seek to promote the interests of the individual patient and the public in general. A professional should always be able to justify any action taken. The midwife is further guided by the 'Midwives rules and code of Practice' (UKCC 1998), which defines her role and remit of practice.

Doctors must also recognise their professional accountability and, in the UK, this has been redefined and presented in the government's white paper *The New NHS: Modern, Dependable* (DOH 1997). This document introduced the concept of Clinical Governance through which trusts have a responsibility to ensure quality of clinical care through the implementation of risk management systems, evidence-based practice, lifelong learning and the systematic audit of clinical performance. Such activities are no longer optional but mandatory.

Legal accountability

Professionals involved in the care of patients have a legal duty to care for them properly, that is to the standard of a reasonable, competent member of that profession (the Bolam test). Failure to do so could result in a patient suing for compensation. In order for a person suing for compensation (the plaintiff) to be awarded damages in respect of negligent care it is their responsibility to demonstrate all of the following:

- The defendant owed a duty of care.
- The defendant was in breach of that duty of care.
- That the damage caused was a direct result of that breach.

It must be noted that *ignorance of the law* is no defence.

Duty of care

The duty of care is clearly established between a health professional and the client. It consists of those elements that constitute treatment, information giving, planning and evaluating care, documentation, supervision and ensuring a safe environment.

Breach of duty

The level at which care should be delivered has been determined through application of the Bolam test. This standard requires that professionals act in a similar manner to a colleague of equivalent status, no higher, no lower. However, where the midwife has assumed the duty of a paediatrician, where she undertakes that duty she should do so with the same skill as the person who would ordinarily perform it. On assuming that responsibility, the nurse or midwife would not be able to say, 'It was my first week' if she made a mistake, but should perform it at the same level as the person who normally undertakes it.

Causation

This is probably the most difficult element of establishing negligence. Even when a condition had failed to be diagnosed, it will only constitute negligence if correct diagnosis would have altered the management of care.

Symon (1998) outlines a case whereby a child had congenital cataracts, which were not diagnosed during the first examination of the newborn. However, an ophthalmologist involved in the case, stated that if the condition had been detected at birth it would have made little difference to the treatment of the child as the prognosis for unilateral cataracts is extremely poor. This is not to suggest that failing to diagnose a condition is without reproach; however, it is not necessarily evidence of negligence, although failure to instigate steps to investigate a condition may be in some circumstances (Symon 1997a). Under current UK law, however, the plaintiff must show causal association between the breach of the practitioner's duty of care and the condition for which damages are being pursued.

It would be appropriate at this point to refer back to the question raised at the beginning of the chapter and apply the three principles of negligent care.

> What is the legal position of a practitioner who does not detect a congenital condition in a baby during the first examination of the newborn?

THE DEFENDANT OWED A DUTY OF CARE

Clearly, by undertaking a professional role, practitioners owe a duty of care to their clients.

BREACH OF THE DUTY OF CARE

A practitioner would be in breach of the duty of care if:

1 They did not gain informed consent from the parents.
2 They failed to take steps to identify it.
3 They were not using commonly accepted techniques to examine the baby.
4 A colleague of equivalent status would have been expected to detect it.
5 They failed to act on a suspicion of abnormality.
6 They did not document their findings.
7 They did not communicate their findings to the parents.
8 They did not follow up investigations requested.

It is clear from this list, that there are many ways in which a practitioner could breach her duty of care to a client, even if she was clinically competent. It is important to ensure that none of the above apply to *your* practice. Failure to detect an abnormality that a colleague of equivalent status would also have missed does not constitute negligence.

CAUSATION

In order to gain compensation for a condition that was not detected at the first examination, the parents would be obliged to prove that detecting it earlier would have made a difference to the outcome.

Employment

Practitioners have a contractual obligation to abide by the policies of the trust which employs them and to take due care in the performance of their duties. The employer has a responsibility to ensure that there are safe systems in place to protect its employees from harm, such as protective clothing.

Trusts will accept liability for the actions of employees during the course of their contracted work and will therefore meet the financial costs of litigation. This is known as *vicarious liability*. It is for this reason that it is usually the trust that is named in negligence cases, even if the trust was not negligent in its duties. If the employee were negligent, the employee would be in breach of the contract of employment, and in law the employer would have the right to be indemnified, although this is unlikely to be pursued.

When a claim for compensation is made

Despite effective clinical care of the mother and her baby, if a congenital abnormality is identified there is a small but real possibility that parents will commence legal action.

> Clinical competence alone will not prevent claims being brought if the outcome is poor.
>
> (Capstick 1993: 10.)

Parents often feel that they must do something positive for the child. It is a terrible fact for parents to face when an abnormality is discovered in a child. There is often a degree of self-blame, and in an attempt to assuage that feeling of guilt parents try to do everything left in their power to alleviate their child's suffering. Making a legal claim for compensation is one way that this phenomenon is manifested.

It is worth bearing in mind that, in England, a change in the legal aid rules in 1990 means that all claims on behalf of infants are funded by the state. Even if the practitioner was not negligent in her duties it is possible that parents, who are distressed because their baby has an abnormality, will file a claim, and the money is available to fund it. It is therefore important that there are no loopholes for the litigant's lawyer to exploit.

The legal process can be a long and protracted affair, with delays occurring at any stage along the way. The time taken from the initial request from the plaintiff's solicitor to see the case notes to a case going to court can be many years.

Although the financial cost of litigation, in terms of compensation, professional time and legal fees, is considerable the human cost of the anguish experienced by the individuals involved in the case is immeasurable. It must be acknowledged, therefore, that action that reduces the risk of negligence claims being filed is time well spent.

The next section focuses on how the effectiveness of the neonatal examination can be enhanced in order to ensure that families receive quality care.

Achieving and maintaining best practice

Practitioners responsible for examination of the newborn should consider the following issues in relation to their role:

1 competence
2 multidisciplinary policy

3 informed consent
4 senior professional and clinical support
5 documentation
6 systematic audit of practice.

Competence

Doctors, nurse and midwives need to address two aspects of their clinical competence to undertake the examination of the newborn: gaining competence and maintaining competence.

Gaining competence

Paediatricians who undertake the examination of the newborn are usually qualified doctors who are working for a paediatric consultant for approximately 6 months. They may go on to specialise in paediatrics or family medicine or, alternatively, use their experience to complement a career in obstetrics. A doctor undertaking this role will therefore already have considerable skill auscultating the heart, listening to the chest and palpating the abdomen in adults. The additional expertise required in order to care for babies will be gained by working alongside senior colleagues, caring for sick neonates and through personal study.

For midwives and nurses to gain the extra skills in order to be competent to perform the full examination of the newborn, it is necessary for them to undertake a post-registration programme of study that exposes the practitioner to this new sphere of practice. This education combines theory with practice and is currently available in the United Kingdom as a recognised course, originally pioneered by Stephanie Michaelides (1995). A senior paediatrician assesses clinical competence, and on successful completion of the course the midwife is able to practice the new skill within the remit of the local policy and trust guidelines. As more nurses and midwives become skilled and experienced in this clinical examination, they will be able to assess the competence of their peers.

Maintaining competence

The Code of Professional Conduct (UKCC 1992, par 3), which both nurses and midwives must abide by, states that as a registered professional, the practitioner must 'maintain and improve professional knowledge and competence'. According to the midwives code of practice (UKCC 1998):

You are responsible for maintaining and developing the competence you have acquired during your initial and subsequent midwifery education.

(UKCC 1998: 28, para 3)

It is central to the practice of all health professionals that they acknowledge the limits of their own individual competence. It is important that practitioners do not run the risk of continuing to care when they are out of their clinical depth by thinking 'I ought to know this' and not seeking advice from senior colleagues because they are too embarrassed to admit that they do not know. It is difficult for senior professionals, who are often seen as the font of all knowledge, to admit to not knowing something, but it would be much more difficult do the same in court. The remit for nurses and midwives is clearly stated in their code of conduct and they must:

…Acknowledge any limitations in your knowledge and competence and decline any duties or responsibilities unless able to perform them in a safe and competent manner.

(UKCC 1992: para 4)

Nurses and midwives are in the fortunate position of usually staying within their speciality for a substantial length of time, thus being able to continue to build on their knowledge and expertise, which junior doctors who are moving between departments every 6 months do not have the luxury of (Denner 1995).

Multidisciplinary policy

The first examination of the newborn is not currently part of the role of all midwives or neonatal nurses. It is essential, therefore, that the midwife or nurse is supported in this expansion of her role by a locally agreed policy that clearly sets out the limits and provides clear guidelines for referral to a paediatrician when support or guidance are required.

The process of sitting down together with fellow colleagues to construct a multidisciplinary policy is an extremely valuable one. Each professional group will gain insight into the constraints and obligations of their respective roles, and this will enhance their future working relationship.

An *example* of such a policy might include the following;

Neonatal examination by a nurse or midwife (practitioner)

Introduction

Examination of the newborn is performed on all babies within the first 24 hours of life. It is currently performed by paediatric senior house officers, general practitioners and, increasingly, midwives and neonatal nurses. Its purpose is to exclude major congenital abnormality and reassure the parents that their baby is healthy. As the length of postnatal stay in hospital is declining, this first examination is often combined with the traditional discharge examination by the doctor and confirms the baby's fitness to go home. It is, therefore, an important screening procedure and health promotion opportunity.

Since the publication of the document *Changing Childbirth* (DOH 1993a) midwives are exploring ways that enable them to provide continuity of care to women and their families. Midwives, without medical input, transfer fit and healthy women to community care. Many midwives feel that after receiving the appropriate education and clinical experience they are best placed to transfer the care of babies into the community.

Aim

To provide parents with the opportunity to have their baby examined by a neonatal nurse or midwife who is competent in this role.

Objectives

The practitioner will

- have a minimum of 2 years of post-registration experience;
- have successfully completed a course of preparation; and
- have access to 24-hour senior paediatric support in the event of an abnormality being either detected or suspected.

Protocol

The practitioner will

- undertake the examination within the first 24 hours of the baby's birth;
- obtain informed consent from a parent;
- undertake examinations on babies that are term, singletons with no known or expected anomalies;
- undertake a full medical examination of the baby in the presence of a parent informed by knowledge of the obstetric, medical and family history;
- make detailed records of the examination in the appropriate case notes;
- record any deviation from normal and inform the paediatrician, informing parents of all findings;
- decline to undertake an examination of a baby when workload pressures or other such circumstances would prevent the examination receiving the attention it requires. In such circumstances the paediatrician or general practitioner would be requested to undertake the examination.

Reviewed by: (senior nurse/midwife/paediatrician)

Review date:

The practitioner could also use the opportunity to draw together an information leaflet for parents outlining the focus of the first examination of their baby, thus making a contribution to the problem of gaining 'informed consent'.

Informed consent

Although the examination of the newborn is a clinical examination that is routinely performed on all day-old babies, consent is still required from the parents before it can be undertaken. In the context of the examination of the newborn the practitioner needs to be aware of both the legal and the professional aspects of gaining consent.

Legal aspects of gaining consent

We have already seen that professionals have a duty of care to provide information to patients, without which they are unable to make an informed choice. Ideally this information should be made available to women before they have to make a decision, so that there is opportunity for them to ask questions and raise concerns. Unfortunately, it is often the case, particularly with non-invasive tests such as ultrasound scanning, that little information is given prior to the event, if at all. Parents are likely to be devastated if their previously 'normal' baby is suddenly found to have a life-threatening abnormality, the diagnosis of which could have been initiated by the neonatal examination. Of course, it would be inappropriate to attempt to prepare every parent for the possibility that a major defect will be detected, but they should know that it is a screening procedure.

It must also be acknowledged that failure to gain consent from the parents to undertake the examination of their baby could also be seen as assault in legal terms. It is also essential that the designation of the practitioner is made clear to parents. If a parent expects a procedure to be undertaken by a doctor, and has no reason to believe that it is not being undertaken by a doctor, then consent may be invalid if the procedure were then undertaken by a nurse or midwife (Martin 1997).

Professional aspects of gaining consent

Maternity services are increasingly endeavouring to offer choices to women regarding the type of care they receive following the recommendations of the document 'Changing Childbirth' (DOH 1993a). In order to make choices, however, women need access to relevant, unbiased information in a language that is meaningful to them. Parents will need to know who you are, the options available, what you are going to do and advantages and disadvantages of the procedure.

Who are you?

Your status and evidence of this should be clearly given to parents. Many professionals do not wear a uniform and this can be confusing for parents. The fear of abduction of babies from maternity units is a real one, and for this reason you should not attempt to remove the baby from the mother's side. Where conditions are not conducive to a personal and thorough examination of the baby, parents should accompany you to a more private location. If you are a nurse or a midwife, you should inform them that you have undertaken further education and supervised practice in order to undertake this role (Dowling *et al.* 1996).

Options available

Depending on the model of care that is operating within the maternity unit, parents should be able to choose to see either a doctor, a nurse or a midwife, without being put under pressure to make a choice. As a nurse or a midwife it would be very easy to say 'you can see a doctor but you will have to wait because they are very busy on the special care baby unit, but I could see you now'. On the other hand, parents do have a right to know the facts, so it might be more appropriate to say, 'you are welcome to see a doctor if you would prefer, and I will find out for you when he or she will be available'. The reality is that most parents will opt to do what everyone else is doing, but their choice of practitioner should be a real one.

What are you going to do?

The purpose and content of the examination should be clearly outlined to the parents. They should be reassured that any significant findings will be discussed with them and that they are free to ask questions during the examination. Failing to communicate effectively is one of the most frequent complaints in health care (DOH 1994).

Advantages and disadvantages of the procedure

This is a very important aspect of gaining informed consent for a procedure. Examination of the newborn is a screening test and as such should be presented in the light of its ability to detect abnormality. Parents need to be aware that although the examination of their baby can exclude conditions such as congenital cataracts it may not detect some forms of heart disease (MacKeith 1995). The converse is also true: where a lax hip joint is detected during this initial examination, it may not be evident subsequently.

Senior professional and clinical support

During the course of professional practice, in every field of health care, there will be the need to consult an expert or seek a second opinion regarding a particular clinical situation. Multidisciplinary team work is vital in the provision of effective, quality care for the family unit. Examining the neonate is such a situation where sometimes confirmation of an observation, such as a suspected heart murmur, is required in order to ensure that the appropriate care is given. It must therefore be ensured that where a practitioner is responsible for examining a neonate that senior paediatric support is available for advice and guidance when needed. This should be clearly documented in the protocol that the practitioner works within so that there is no confusion about who that clinician might be at any given time.

Professional support is also required so that the practitioner can discuss any issues pertaining to practice, such as continuing professional development and workload pressures. In midwifery, the practitioner can approach the supervisor of midwives for support and guidance. The practising midwife has 24-hour access to a supervisor of midwives, who can offer advice and information enabling the midwife to continue to provide quality care. The remit of the supervisor of midwives is to safeguard the mother and her baby by ensuring that midwives are able to maintain and develop their professional knowledge while acknowledging the limits of their competence. Increasingly in nursing, clinical supervision is a mechanism that enables the practitioner to reflect on professional and practice issues (Cowe and Wilkes 1998). Supervisors are optimally placed to understand the unique culture of the organisation in which the practitioner is working and therefore be empathetic to her needs. Practitioners should meet regularly with their supervisors not only for professional support, but also to discuss and evaluate their roles within ever evolving health services.

Documentation

Records are a vital way in which health care professionals communicate with each other. The nature of health care work is such that we see many patients each day in similar circumstances, but requiring individualised care. Records help ensure that observations are communicated to colleagues, including any subsequent action taken, who was involved and when. Many maternity records are patient-held and therefore the parents may have access to this information in the comfort of their own home. Just because the parents do not have a medical or legal background does not mean that their friends and relatives do not. There are some basic requirements that help make records effective:

- Do not use abbreviations unless a standard list of locally approved abbreviations accompanies each set of records. Abbreviations are open to misinterpretation and can lead to mistakes being made.
- Always date, time and sign each entry, stating your designation at least once on the record.
- Always write in black as it photocopies much more clearly should a copy be required.
- If you have requested referral, further tests or investigations ensure that they are documented and evaluated. All actions taken and advice given should be clearly written.
- It is also relevant to document circumstances that may have contributed to an inability to perform the examination adequately. Such an entry must be accompanied by a plan to deal with the situation. Table 7.1 illustrates how this might apply in practice.
- If unavoidable circumstances had prevented the practitioner from returning to the baby, the situation should be explained to the mother and alternative arrangements made and documented in the case notes.
- Do not make amendments to records with correction fluid, but if necessary score a single line throughout the text so that what is written underneath can be clearly read, write 'written in error' and sign the entry.
- Where possible use language that is clear and accessible to the client so that it can be read with a minimum of translation. This will avoid confusion and fear caused by the use of jargon and technical language. Records should be written bearing in mind that the patients have access to all written records about themselves which were made after November 1991 (Access to Health Records Act 1990). They should therefore not contain any material which might be subjective, offensive or irrelevant. In ideal circumstances records should be made in front of patients so that they have a full knowledge of what observations have been documented.

It cannot be emphasised too strongly how important clear, concise records are; further detail is provided in the document 'Guidelines for Records and Record Keeping' (UKCC 1998a). Excellence in record keeping is central to proactive risk management. The existence of accurate, contemporaneous records may actually prevent a case ever coming to court. If a plaintiff's solicitor writes to the hospital trust outlining a possible claim and asking for the case notes to be disclosed,

TABLE 7.1 An example of a written entry in the notes

Date/time	Record	Signature	Designation
10.40	Unable to auscultate the heart as baby Smith was crying Plan: repeat examination this afternoon. Mother and Midwife Jones informed	*Helen Baston*	Midwife
15.20	Baby Smith calm and re-examined Normal heart sounds heard. Mother informed, fit for transfer	*Helen Baston*	Midwife

this is when cases are often either thrown out or pursued. There is a professional duty to keep such records and failure to do so may lead to the assumption that the care also failed to come up to scratch. A useful aspect to bear in mind when considering record keeping is the maxim that 'if it is not documented it did not happen'.

Detailed patient records are an investment for the future because the child who is damaged in the perinatal period has up to 21 years in which to file a claim; there is no time limit for a child who is deemed incapable of managing their own affairs (Capstick 1993). Accurate records are therefore invaluable as many staff have difficulties recollecting a particular case (Symon 1997b). We cannot see into the future and predict which parents will file for negligence on behalf of their child. It would be almost impossible to remember the precise details of what actions were taken or what referrals were made many years after the event. Although it may seem tedious at the time to make detailed notes of such interactions, if a case were brought to court these records would form an essential part of the defence.

It has been shown how clear, accurate and detailed records can assist the delivery of quality care and also act in a practitioners defence should a negligence case be initiated.

Systematic audit of practice

Audit is 'the systematic and critical analysis of the quality of clinical

TABLE 7.2 Donabedian's dimensions of quality

Criteria	Characteristics	Example in practice
Structure	Resources required	Policies, skills, equipment
Process	Actions undertaken	Gaining consent, documentation, examination
Outcome	Desired effect	Patient satisfaction, no detectable abnormalities missed

care' (DOH 1993b), and through the implementation of clinical governance in the National Health Service in the UK it is an integral part of health care provision (DOH 1997). Audit involves identifying what is best practice, setting standards and then comparing practice against those standards. It is a dynamic process through which changes can be recommended and then subsequent care re-audited, and thus the cycle continues.

There are many aspects of the examination of the newborn process that can be audited in order to ensure that quality of care is continually improved.

Donabedian (1966) suggested three aspects of care that, through their examination, can assist the practitioner to enhance quality issues. These are: structure, process and outcome (see Table 7.2).

Audit involves change, and it is therefore important that the people who the change would effect are involved at the beginning of any audit project. Planning should include all members of the multidisciplinary team and managers who might be responsible for implementing any of the recommendations.

Conclusion

This chapter has given readers an insight into how their professional and legal accountability affect their role when undertaking the first examination of the newborn. There are many ways in which the practitioner can enhance the effectiveness of the examination, thus minimising the risk of mistakes being made and negligence suits being filed.

It is a privilege to be with women and their families at this special time in their lives. Every possible care should be taken to ensure that as health care professionals, we make a positive contribution to the experience of the birth of their baby.

Appendix 1

Useful addresses

Action on Smoking and Health (ASH)
5/11 Mortimer Street, London W1N 7RH
Tel: 020 7637 9843   Fax: 020 7436 4750

Alcoholics Anonymous
PO Box 1, Stonebow House, Stonebow, York YO1 2NJ
Tel: 01904 644026

Association for Children with Hand or Arm Deficiency (REACH)
12, Wilson Way, Earls Barton, Northamptonshire, NN6 0NZ
Tel: 01604 811041   Fax: 01604 811041

Association for Improvements in Maternity Services (AIMS)
40 Kingswood Avenue, London, NW6 6IS
Tel: 020 8960 5585   Fax: 01753 654142

Association for Spina Bifida and Hydrocephalus (ASBAH)
42 Park Road, Peterborough, Cambs PE1 2UQ
Tel: 01733 555988   Fax: 01733 555985
E-mail: rosemaryb@asbah.demon.co.uk

Baby Life Support Systems (BLISS)
17–21 Emerald Street, London WC1N 3QL
Tel: 020 7831 9393   Fax: 020 7404 0676

Body Positive
51B Philbeach Gardens, London SW5 9EB
Tel: 020 7835 1045
Fax: 020 7373 5237

British Institute for Brain Injured Children
Knowle Hall, Knowle, Bridgwater, Somerset, TA7 8PJ
Tel 01278 684060   Fax: 01278 685573

British Heart Foundation
102 Gloucester Place, London, W1H 4DH
Tel: 020 79350185

British Diabetic Association
10 Queen Anne Street, London W1M 0BD
Tel: 020 76366112   Fax: 020 76373644
E-mail: BDA@BBCNC.ORG.Uk

British Pregnancy Advisory Service
Austy Manor, Wooton Wawen, Solihull, West Midlands B95 6BX
Tel: 01564 793225   Fax: 01564 794935

Brook Advisory Centres
165 Grays Inn Road, London WC1X 8UD
Tel: 020 7833 8488   Fax: 020 7833 8182

Caesarean Support Network
55 Cooil Drive, Douglas, Isle of Man IM2 2HF
Tel: 01624 661269

Cleft Lip and Palate Association (CLAPA)
134 Buckingham Palace Road, London SW1 9SA
Tel: 020 7824 8110   Fax: 020 7824 8109

Cry-sis
B.M. Cry-sis, London WC1N 3XX
Tel: 01634 710913   Fax: 01634 710913

Cystic Fibrosis Research Trust
Alexandra House, 5 Blyth Road, Bromley, Kent BR1 3RS
Tel: 020 8464 7211   Fax: 020 8313 0472

Cystic Hygroma and Haemangioma Support Group (CHHSG)
Villa Fontane, Church Road, Worth, Crawly, West Sussex RH10 4RS
Tel: 01293 885901   Fax: 01293 882460

Disfigurement Guidance Centre
PO Box 7, Cupar, Fife KY15 4PF
Tel: 01337 870281   Fax: 01337 870 310

Down's Syndrome Association
155 Mitcham Road, Tooting, London SW17 9PG
Tel: 020 86824001   Fax: 020 86824012

Drugline
9a Brockley Cross, Brockley, London SE4 2AB
Tel: 020 86924975

Dystrophic Epidermolysis Bullosa Research Association (DEBRA)
Debra House, 13 Wellington Business Park, Dukes Ride,
Crowthorne RG45 6LS
Tel: 01344 771961   Fax: 01344 762661

Foresight: Association for the Promotion of Preconceptual Care
28 The Paddock, Godalming, Surrey GU7 1XD
Tel: 01483 427839   Fax: 01483 427668

Foundation for the Study of Infant Deaths
14 Halkin Street, London SW1X 7DP
Tel: 020 72350965   Fax: 020 78231986

Gingerbread (Association for one parent families)
16/17 Clerkenwell Close London EC1R 0AA
Tel 020 73368183   Fax: 020 73368185
E-mail:ginger@lonepar.demon.co.uk

Herpes Viruses Association (HVA SPHERE)
41 North Road, London N7 9DP
Tel: 020 76079661

Hospice Information
St Christopher's Hospice, 51–59 Lawrie Park Road, Sydenham,
London SE26 6DZ
Tel: 020 87789252

La Leche League of Great Britain
BM 3424, London WC1V 6XX
Tel: 020 72421278

MAMA Meet a Mum Association
Cornerstone House, 14 Willis Road, Croydon, Surrey CR0 2XX
Tel 020 86650357   Fax: 020 86651972

Maternity Alliance
45, Beech Street, London EC2P 2LX
Tel: 020 75888583   Fax: 020 75888584

Naevus (Birthmark) Support Group
58 Necton Road, Wheathampstead, Herts AL4 8AU
Tel: 01582 832853

**(STEPS) National Association for Families of Children with
Congenital Abnormalities of the Lower Limbs**
15, Statham Close, Lymm, Cheshire WA13 9NN
Tel: 01925 757525   Fax: 01925 757525
E-mail: steps@itl.net

National Childbirth Trust
Alexandra House, Oldham Terrace, Acton, London W3 6NH
Tel 020 89922616   Fax: 020 89925929

National Deaf–Blind and Rubella Association (SENSE)
11–13 Clifton Terrace, Finsbury Park, London N4 3SR
Tel: 020 72727774   Fax 020 72726012

National Eczema Society (NES)
163 Eversholt Street, London NW1 1BU
Tel: 020 7388 4800   Fax: 020 73885882

National Meningitis Trust
Fern House, Bath Road, Stroud, Glos GL5 3TJ
Tel: 01453 751738   Fax: 01453 753588

National Stepfamily Association
3rd Floor, Chapel House, 18 Hatton Place, London EC1N 8RU
Tel: 0990 168388   Fax: 020 72092461

Parentline
Endway House, The Endway, Hadleigh, Essex SS7 2AN
Tel: 01702 554782   Fax: 01702 554911

Pre-eclamptic Toxaemia Society (PETS)
12 Monksford Drive, Hullbridge, Hockley, Essex SS5 6DQ
Tel: 01702 230493

Royal National Institute for Deaf People (RNID)
19–23 Featherstone Street, London EC1Y 8SL
Tel: 020 72968000   Fax: 020 72968199

Royal National Institute for the Blind (RNIB)
224 Great Portland Street, London W1N 6AA
Tel: 020 73881266   Fax 020 73882034
E-mail: rnib@rnib.org.uk

Samaritans
17 Uxbridge Road, Slough SL1 1SN
Tel: 01753 32713   Fax: 01753 24322

Sickle Cell Society
54 Station Road, Harlesden, London NW10 4UA
Tel: 020 89617795   Fax: 020 89618346

SCOPE
12 Park Crescent, London W1N 4EQ
Tel: 020 76365020   Fax: 020 74362601

Stillbirth and Neonatal Death Society (SANDS)
28 Portland Place, London W1N 4DE
Tel: 020 74365881   Fax: 020 74363715

Terrence Higgins Trust
52–54 Grays Inn Road, London WC1X 8JU
Tel: 020 7831 0330   Fax: 020 78164552
E-mail: info@tht.org.uk

Twins and Multiple Births Association
PO Box 30, Little Sutton, South Wirral L66 1TH
Tel: 0151 3480020   Fax: 0151 2005309

Appendix 2

Safe sleeping environment for babies: advice for parents

- Smoke-free
- Room temperature approximately 18°C
- Lie baby on its back
- Do not wedge baby on its side
- Do not overwrap baby
- Use several thin layers of blankets
- Do not use pillow or duvet
- Lie baby with its 'feet to foot' of the cot
- Ensure no loose ties on clothes/toys
- No flexes/mobiles within reach of crib
- Keep animals out of room
- Install smoke detector

Note
For further information contact the Foundation for the Study of Infant Death (FSID),
14 Halkin Street, London SW1X 7DP
24-hour helpline: 020 7235 1721

References

Access to Health Records Act (1990) HMSO: London.

ACOG Technical Bulletin (1993) Perinatal viral and parasitic infections. *International Journal of Gynaecology and Obstetrics* 42(177): 300–7.

Adhikari M, Gouws E, Velaphi SC, Gwamanda P. (1998) Meconium aspiration syndrome: importance of the monitoring of labour. *Journal of Perinatology* 18(1): 55–60.

Adra AM, Mejides AA, Dennaoui MS, Beydoun SN (1995) Fetal pyelectasis: is it always 'physiologic'? *American Journal of Obstetrics and Gynaecology* 173(4):1263–6.

Akhter MS (1976) An unusual complication of intrapartum fetal monitoring. *American Journal of Obstetrics and Gynaecology* 15: 657–8.

Alcock KM (1992) Teenage pregnancy and sex education. *British Journal of Family Planning* 18(3): 88–92.

Alderice F, Renfrew M, Marchant S, Ashurst H, Hughes P, Berridge G, Garcia JI (1995) Labour and birth in England and Wales: survey report. *British Journal of Midwifery* 3(7): 375–82.

Alexander JM, Cox SM (1996) Clinical course of premature rupture of the membranes. *Seminars in Perinatology* 20(5): 369–74.

Allott H (1996) Picking up the pieces: the post-delivery stress clinic. *British Journal of Midwifery* 4(10): 534–6.

Alroomi LG (1988) Maternal narcotic abuse and the newborn. *Archives of Diseases in Childhood* 63(1): 81–3.

Armant DR, Suanders DE (1996) Exposure of embryonic cells to alcohol: contrasting effects during preimplantation development. *Seminars in Perinatology* 20(2): 127–39.

Bardy AH, Seppala T, Lillsunde P, Kataja JM, Koskela P, Pikkarainen J, Hiilesmaa VK (1993) Objectively measured tobacco exposure during pregnancy: neonatal effects and relation to maternal smoking. *British Journal of Obstetrics and Gynaecology* 100: 721–6.

Beal SM, Byard RW (1995) Accidental death or sudden infant death syndrome? *Journal of Paediatric Child Health* 31(4): 269–71.

Beckwith J, Read M (1996) Prelabour rupture of membranes at term: home management. *British Journal of Midwifery* 4(2): 74–5.

Bennett VK, Brown LK (eds) (1999) *Myles Textbook for Midwives*, 13th edn. Churchill Livingstone: London.

Boivin JF (1997) Risk of spontaneous abortion in women occupationally exposed to anaesthetic gases: a meta-analysis. *Occupational Environmental Medicine* 54(8): 541–8.

Bowlby J (1953) *Child Care and the Growth of Love.* Penguin: London.

Brown L (1998) The tide has turned audit of water birth. *British Journal of Midwifery* 6(4): 236–43.

Butler N, Ineichen B, Taylor B, Wandsworth J (1981) *Teenage Mothering.* 2. Report to DHSS, University of Bristol: Bristol.

Butler NR, *et al.* (1972) Cigarette smoking in pregnancy: its influence on birthweight and perinatal mortality. *British Medical Journal* 15: 127–30.

Campbell MK (1998) Factors affecting outcome in post-term birth. *Current Opinion in Obstetrics and Gynaecology* 9(6): 356–60.

Campion P, Owen L, McNeill A, McGuire C (1994) Evaluation of a mass media campaign on smoking and pregnancy. *Addiction* 89: 1245–54.

Capstick B (ed.) (1993) *Litigation. A risk Management Guide for Midwives.* The Royal College of Midwives: Kent.

Carbonne B, Langer B, Goffinet F, Audibert F, Tardif D, Le Goueff F, Laville M, Maillard F (1997) Multicenter study on the clinical value of fetal pulse oximetry. II. Compared predictive values of pulse oximetry and fetal blood analysis. The French Study Group on Fetal Pulse Oximetry. *American Journal of Obstetrics and Gynaecology.* 177(3): 593–8.

Chalmers JA, Chalmers I (1989) The obstetric vacuum extractor is the instrument of first choice for operative vaginal delivery. *British Journal of Obstetrics and Gynaecology* 98: 505–9.

Chan A, McCaul KA, Cundy PJ, Haan EA, Byron-Scott R (1997) Perinatal risk factors for developmental dysplasia of the hip. *Archives of Disease in Childhood* 76(2): F94–F100.

Chaplin J, McDiarmid P (1992) Teenage parenthood – myth and reality. *Community Health Action* 25(Autumn): 3.

Chattingius S, Haglund B (1997) Decreasing smoking prevalence during pregnancy in Sweden: the effect on small for gestational age births. *American Journal of Public Health* 87(3): 410–3.

Chen ZL (1992) A case–control study on the relationship between neonatal hyperbilirubaemia and usage of oxytocin during labour. *Chung Hua Hsing Ping Hsueh Tsa Chih* 13(5):294–6.

Chew S, Anandakumar C, Wong YC (1995) Fetal choroid plexus cysts and their association with aneuploidy. *Journal of Obstetrics and Gynaecology* 15(6): 359–62.

Corson SL (1998) Achieving and maintaining pregnancy after age 40. *International Journal of Fertility and Womens Medicine* 43(5): 249–56.

Cowe F, Wilkes C (1998) Clinical supervision for specialist nurses. *Professional Nurse* 13(5): 284–7.

Crang-Svalenius E, Dykes AK, Jorgensen C (1996) Organised routine ultrasound in the second trimester. One hundred womens experiences. *Journal of Maternal-Fetal Investigation* 6(4): 219–22.

Crompton J (1996) Post-traumatic stress disorder and childbirth. *British Journal of Midwifery* 4(6): 290–5.

Denner S (1995) Extending professional practice: benefits and pitfalls. *Nursing Times* 91(14): 27–9.

Department of Health (1993a) *Changing Childbirth.* HMSO: London

Department of Health (1993b) *Clinical Audit. Meeting and improving standards in health care.* The Health Publications Unit: Heywood, UK.

Department of Health (1994) *Being Heard: The Report of a Review Committee on NHS Complaints Procedures*. HMSO: London.

Department of Health (1997) *The New NHS: Modern, Dependable*. HMSO: London.

Divon MY, Haglund B, Nisell ER, Otterblad PO, Westgren M (1998) Fetal and neonatal mortality in the postterm pregnancy: the impact of gestational age and fetal growth restriction. *American Journal of Obstetrics and Gynaecology* 178(4): 726–31.

Donabedian A (1966) Evaluating the quality of medical Care. *Millbank Memorial Fund* 44(3) (Suppl): 166–206.

Donnenfeld AE (1995) Prenatal sonographic detection of isolated fetal choroid plexus cysts: should we screen for trisomy 18? *Journal of Medical Screening* 2(1): 18–21.

Dowling S, Martin R, Skidmore P, Doyal L, Cameron A, Lloyd S (1996) Nurses taking on junior doctors work: a confusion of accountability. *British Medical Journal* 312: 1211–14.

Drugs and Therapeutic Bulletin (1997) Managing post-term pregnancy. *Drugs and Therapeutics Bulletin* 35(3): 17–18.

Duncan G, *et al.* (1990) Termination of pregnancy: lessons for prevention. *British Journal of Family Planning* 15: 112–17.

English DR, Hulse GK, Milne E, Holman CD, Bower CI (1997) Maternal cannabis use and low birth weight: a meta-analysis. *Addiction* 92(11): 1553–60.

Enkin MW, Keirse MJNC, Renfrew MJ, Neilson JP (eds) (1995) *Pregnancy and Childbirth Module of the Cochrane Database of Systematic Reviews*. BMJ Publishing: London.

FIGO (1984) Report of the FIGO subcommittee on perinatal epidemiology and health statistics following a workshop in Cairo November 11–18 on the methodology of measurement and recording of infant growth in the perinatal period. FIGO London: 54. In Alfirevic Z, Walkinshaw SA. (1994).

Fisch B, Harel L, Kaplan B, Pinkas H, Amit S, Ovadia J, Tadir Y, Merlob P (1997) Neonatal assessment of babies conceived by in vitro fertilisation. *Journal of Perinatology* 17(6): 473–6.

Florey C, Taylor D, Blumaar F (eds) (1992) EUROMAC. A European concentrated action: maternal alcohol consumption and its relation to the outcome of pregnancy and child development at eighteen months. *International Journal of Epidemiology*, 21(4): Suppl 1.

Ford RPK, Tappin DM, Schluter PJ, Wild CJ (1997) Smoking during pregnancy: how reliable are maternal self reports in New Zealand? *Journal of Epidemiology and Community Health* 51(3): 246–51.

Foresight Association for the Promotion of Pre-conceptual Care. (1996) *Foresight Easter Newsletter*. Europress.

Freeborn SF, Calvert RT, Black P (1980) Saliva and blood pethidine concentrations in the mother and newborn baby. *British Journal of Obstetrics and Gynaecology* 87: 966–9.

Gamsu H (1993) The effects of pain relief on the baby. In Chamberlain G, Wraight A, Steer P (eds) *Pain and its Relief in Childbirth*. Churchill Livingstone: Edinburgh.

Geary M, Crowley D, Boylan P (1997) Passive cigarette smoking in pregnancy. *Journal of Obstetrics and Gynaecology* 17(3): 264–5.

Gersovich EO (1997) A radiologist's guide to the imaging in the diagnosis and treatment of developmental dysplasia of the hip. General Considerations, phyusical examination as applied to real time sonography and radiography. *Skeletal Radiology* 26(7): 386–97.

Gilbert WM, Nesbitt TS, Danielsen B (1999) Childbearing beyond age 40: pregnancy outcome in 24,032 cases. *Obstetrics and Gynaecology* 93(1): 9–14.

Gillies P, Wakefield M (1993) Smoking in pregnancy. *Current Obstetrics and Gynaecology* 3(3): 157–61.

Green J, Statham H (1993) Testing for abnormality in routine antenatal care. *Midwifery* 9(3): 124–35.

Green JM, Kitzinger JV, Coupland VA (1990) Stereotypes of childbearing women: a look at some evidence. *Midwifery* 6: 125–32.

Gregory J, Emslie A, Wyllie J, Wren C (1999) Examination for cardiac malformations at six weeks of age. *Archives of Disease in Childhood. Fetal and Neonatal Edition* 80(1): F46–8.

Gupta JK, Cave M, Lilford RJ, Farrell TA, Irving HC, Mason G, Hau CM (1995) Clinical significance of fetal choroid plexus cysts. *Lancet* 346(8977): 724–9.

Haglund B, Chattingius S (1990) Cigarette smoking as a risk factor for sudden infant death syndrome, a population based study. *American Journal of Public Health* 80(1): 29–32.

Hall DMB (1996) *Health for all Children*. Oxford University Press: Oxford.

Hall DMB (1999) The role of the routine neonatal examination (Editorial). *British Medical Journal* 318(7184): 19–20.

Hall MH, Chng PK, Macgillivray I (1980) Is antenatal care worthwhile. *Lancet* 2: 78–80.

Hampshire S (1984) *The Maternal Instinct*. Collins: Glasgow.

Hannah ME, Ohlsson A, Farine D, Hewson SA, Hodnett ED, Myhr Tl, Wang EE, Weston JA, Willan AR (1996) Induction of labour compared with expectant management of prelabor rupture of the membranes at term. *New England Journal of Medicine* 334(16): 1005–10.

Haugland S, Haug K, Wold B (1996) A pregnant smokers experience of antenatal care – results from a qualitative study. *Scandinavian Journal of Primary Health Care* 14(4): 216–22.

Haverkamp AD, Orleans M, Langenoerfer, S McFee J, Murphy J (1979) A controlled trial of the different effects of intrapartum fetal monitoring. *American Journal of Obstetrics and Gynaecology* 134(4): 399–412.

Haworth SG, Bull C (1993) Physiology of congenital heart disease. *Archives of Disease in Childhood* 68: 707–11.

Health Education Authority (1996) *Thinking of Having a Baby? Folic Acid – What all Women Should Know*. Health education leaflet. ISBN 0 7521 05787.

Hemminki K, Kyyronen P, Lindbohm ML (1985) Spontaneous abortions and malformations in the offspring of nurses exposed to anaesthetic gases, cytostatic drugs, and other potential hazards in hospitals, based on registered information of outcome. *Journal of Epidemiology and Community Health* 39(2): 141–7.

Hepburn M (1993) Drug misuse in pregnancy. *Current Obstetrics and Gynaecology* 3: 54–8.

Hilder L, Costeloe K, Thiganathan B (1998) Prolonged pregnancy: evaluating gestation specific risks of fetal and infant mortality. *British Journal of Obstetrics and Gynaecology* 105(2): 169–73.

Hilton T (1991) *The Great Ormond Street Book of Baby and Child Care*. BCA: London.

Hull D, Johnston DI (1993) *Essential Paediatrics*, 3rd edn. Churchill Livingstone: Edinburgh.

Human Fertilisation and Embryology Authority (1999) *8th Annual Report and Accounts*. The Stationary Office: UK

Jacob J, Pfenninger J (1997) Cesarean deliveries: when is a paediatrician necessary? *Obstetrics and Gynaecology* 89(2): 217–20.

Jennings SE (ed.) (1995) *Infertility Counselling*. Blackwell Science: Oxford.

Jensen TK, Hjollund NHI, Henriksen TB, Scheike T, Kolstad H, Giwercman A, Ernst E, Bonde JP, Skakkebaek NE, Olsen Jl (1998) Does moderate alcohol consumption affect fertility? Follow-up study among couples planning first pregnancy. *British Medical Journal* 317(7157): 505–10.

Johanson RB, Menon BKV (2000) Vacuum extraction versus forceps for assisted vaginal delivery (Review). The Cochrane Database of Systematic Reviews. *The Cochrane Library* 1(1): 1–14.

Johnson JD, Aldrich M, Angelus P, Stevenson DK, Smith DW, Hersche MJ, Papagaroufalsi C, Valaes T (1984) Oxytocin and neonatal hyperbilirubinaemia. Studies of bilirubin production. *American Journal of Diseases in Childhood* 138(11): 1047–50.

Jolly H (1985) *Hugh Jolly Book of Child care. The Complete Guide for Today's Parents*. Unwin Hyman Limited: London.

Jones KL, Smith DW (1973) Recognition of fetal alcohol syndrome in infancy. *Lancet* 2, 999–1001.

Jones KL (1997) *Smiths Recognizable Patterns of Human Malformation*. WB Saunders Company: Philadelphia.

Jones EF (ed) (1986) *Teenage Pregnancy in Industrialised Countries*. Yale University Press: Newhaven.

Jorgensen FS (1995) User acceptability of an alpha feto-protein screening programme. *Danish Medical Bulletin* 42(1): 100–5.

Katwijk van C, Peeter LL (1998) Clinical aspects of pregnancy after the age of 35 years: a review of the literature. *Human Reproduction Update* 4(2): 185–94.

Kaufman MH (1997) The teratogenic affects of alcohol exposure during pregnancy, and its influence on the chromosome constitution of the pre-ovulatory egg. *Alcohol and Alcoholism* 32(2): 113–28.

Kelso IM, Parsons RJ, Lawrence GF, Arora SS, Edmonds DK, Cooke ID (1978) An assessment of continuous fetal heart rate monitoring in labour: A randomised trial. *American Journal of Obstetrics and Gynaecology* 131(5): 526–32.

Klima CS (1998) Emergency contraception for midwifery practice. *Journal of Nurse-Midwifery* 43(3): 182–9.

Ladfors L, Mattsson LA, Eriksson M, Fall O (1996) A randomised trial of two expectant managements of prelabour rupture of the membranes at 34 to 42 weeks. *British Journal of Obstetrics and Gynaecology* 103: 755–62.

Leslie KK, Persutte WH, Drose JA, Lenke RR, Hobbins JC, Manco-Johnson M, Shaffer E, Wiggins J (1996) Prenatal detection of congenital heart disease by basic ultrasonography at a tertiary care center: what should our expectations be? *Journal of Maternal-Fetal Investigation* 6(3): 132–5.

Lieberman E, Lang JM, Frigoletto F, Acker D, Rao R (1997) Epidural analgesia, intrapartum fever, and neonatal sepsis evaluation. *Pediatrics* 99(3): 415–19.

Lindqvist A, Norden-Lindeberg S, Hanson U (1997) Perinatal mortality and route of delivery in term breech presentations. *British Journal of Obstetrics and Gynaecology* 104(11): 1288–91.

Lissauer TJ, Steer PJ (1988) The relationship between the need for intubation at birth, abnormal cardiotocograms in labour and cord artery blood gas and pH values. *British Journal of Obstetrics and Gynaecology* 93(10): 1060–6.

Luke B (1994) Nutritional influences on fetal growth. *Clinical Obstetrics and Gynaecology* 37(3): 538–49.

MacDonald D, Grant A, Sheridan-Pereira M, Boylan P, Chalmers I (1985) The Dublin randomised controlled trial of intrapartum fetal heart rate monitoring. *American Journal of Obstetrics and Gynaecology* 152(5): 524–39.

McFarlane, Parker B, Soeken K (1996) Physical abuse, smoking, and substance use during pregnancy: prevalence, interrelationships, and effects on birth weight. *Journal of Obstetric, Gynaecological and Neonatal Nursing* 25(4): 313–20.

MacKeith N (1995) Who should examine the normal neonate. *Nursing Times* 91(14): 34–35.

McKenna A, Woolwich C, Burgess K. (1994) The emergency nurse practitioner. In Sbaih L (ed.) *Issues in Accident and Emergency Nursing*. Chapman & Hall: London.

McMahon CA, Ungereer JA, Beaurepaire J, Tennant C, Saunders D (1995) Psychosocial outcomes for parents and children after in vitro fertilisation: a review. *Journal of Reproductive and Infant Psychology* 13: 1–16.

McNamara J (1995) *Bruised Before Birth. Parenting Children Exposed to Parental Substance Abuse*. British Agencies for Adoption and Fostering: London.

Madeley RJ, Gillies PA, Power FL, Symonds EM (1989) Nottingham mothers stop smoking project – baseline survey of smoking in pregnancy. *Community Medicine* 11: 124–30.

Manning FA, Bondaji N, Harman CR, Casiro O, Menticoglou S, Morrison I, Bersk DJ (1998) Fetal assessment based on fetal biophysical profile scoring. VIII. The incidence of cerebral palsy in tested and untested perinates. *American Jouranal of Obstetrics and Gynaecology* 178(4): 696–706.

Martin R (1997) Changing boundaries and legal risk. A challenge for nursing. *Health Care Risk Report* June: 13–15.

Medical Research Council (1991) Prevention of Neural tube defects: results of the medical Research Council Vitamin Study. MRC Vitamin Study Group. *Lancet* July 20, 338, 8760: 131–7.

Mercier FJ, Benhamou D (1997) Hyperthermia related to epidural analgesia during labor. *International Journal of Obstetric Anaesthesia* 6: 19–24.

Michaelides S (1995) A deeper knowledge. *Nursing Times* 91(35): 59–61.

Michaelides S (1997) Newborn examination: whose responsibility? *British Journal of Midwifery* 5(9): 538.

Ministry of Health (1929) 145/MCW.

Myhra W, Davis M, Mueller BA, Hickok D (1992) Maternal smoking and the risk of polyhydramnios. *American Journal of Public Health* 82(2): 176–9.

Myles M (1993) *Text Book for Midwives*, 12th edn. Churchill Livingstone: Edinburgh.

National Infertility Awareness Campaign (1998) *Report of the Sixth National Survey of the Funding and Provision of Infertility Services*. College of Health: London.

Neuspiel DR, Rush D, Butler NR, Golding J, Bijur PE, Kurzon M (1989) Parental smoking and post-infancy wheezing in children: a prospective cohort study. *American Journal of Public Health* 79(2): 168–71.

Nora JG (1990) Perinatal cocaine use: maternal, fetal and neonatal effects. *Neonatal Network* 9(2): 45–52.

Nyagu AL, Loganovsky KN, Loganovskaja TK (1998) Psychophysiologic after effects of prenatal irradiation. *International Journal of Psychophysiology* 30(3): 303–11.

Odent M (1998) Use of water during labour – updated recommendations. *MIDIRS Midwifery Digest* 8(1): 68–9.

Office for National Statistics (1998) *Social Trends 28*. The Stationary Office: London.

Olofsson CH, Ekblom A, Ekman-Ordeberg G, Hjelm A, Irested L (1996) Lack of analgesic effect of systematically administered morphine or pethidine on labour pain. *British Journal of Obstetrics and Gynaecology* 103(10): 968–72.

Ottervanger HP, Keirse MJNC, Smit W, Holm JP (1996) Controlled comparison of induction versus expectant care for prelabour rupture of the membranes at term. *Journal of Prenatal Medicine* 24(3): 237–42.

Pheonix A (1990) *Young Mothers*. Polity Press: Oxford.

Piper JM, Newton ER, Berkus MD, Peairs WA (1998) Meconium: a marker for peripartum infection. *Obstetrics and Gynaecology* 91(5): 741–5.

Pleasure JR, Stahl GE. Do epidural anesthesia-related maternal fevers alter neonatal care? *Pediatric Research* 27: 221.

Plessinger MA (1998) Prenatal exposure to amphetamines. Risks and adverse outcomes in pregnancy. *Obstetrics and Gynaecology Clinics of North America* 25(1): 119–38.

Polin RA, Fox WW (1998) *Fetal and Neonatal Physiology*, vol. 1, 2nd edn. WB Saunders Company: Philadelphia.

Prochaska JO, DiClemente CC (1983) Stages and processes of self-change of smoking: towards an integrative model. *Journal of Consulting and Clinical Psychology* 51: 390–5.

Ramsay CR, Glazener CMA, Campbell MK, Booth P, Duffty P, Lloyd DJ, McDonald A, Reid JA (1997) Neonatal screening examinations: is one examination enough? *Journal of Epidemiology and Community Health* 51(5): 606.

Raphael-Leff J (1991) *Psychological Processes of Childbearing*. Chapman & Hall: London.

Richardson D (1993) *Women, Motherhood and Childrearing*. Macmillan: London.

Roach VJ, Rogers MS (1997) Pregnancy outcome beyond 41 weeks gestation. *International Journal of Gynaecology and Obstetrics* 59(1): 19–24.

Roberton NRC (1986) *A Manual of Neonatal Intensive Care*. Arnold: London.

Roberton NRC (1996) *A Manual of Normal Neonatal Care*, 2nd edn. Arnold: London.

Robinson J (2000) Ultrasound; the slippery slope. *British Journal of Midwifery* 8(1): 24.

Roch S, Alexander J, Levey V (1990) *Postnatal Care. A Research-based Approach*. Macmillan: London.

Rogers J (1997) It could be you. Antenatal screening. *Nursing Times* 93(6): 54–5.

Rothman BK (1988) *The Tentative Pregnancy Prenatal Diagnosis and the Future of Motherhood*. Pandora: London.

Royal College of Obstetricians and Gynaecologists (1997) Alcohol consumption in pregnancy. Press Release RCOG, London.

Royal College of Physicians (1993) *Smoking and the Young*. Royal College of Physicians: London.

Salvesen KA, Bakketeig LS, Eik-nes SH, Undeheim JO, Oakland O (1992) Routine ultrasonography *in utero* and school performance at age 8–9 years. *Lancet* 339(8785): 85–9.

Salvesen KA, Eik-nes SH (1999) Ultrasound during pregnancy and subsequent childhood non-right handedness: a meta-analysis. *Ultrasound in Obstetrics and Gynaecology* 13(4): 241–6.

Sarker PK, Hill L (1996) Maternal anxiety and depression – the experience of prolonged pregnancy. *Journal of Obstetrics and Gynaecology* 16(6): 488–92.

Seidel HM, Rosenstein BJ, Pathak A (1997) *Primary Care of the Newborn*, 2nd edn. Mosby: London.

Sharma JB, Newman MR, Bouttchier JE, Williams A (1997) National audit on the practice and training in breech deliveries in the United Kingdom. *International Journal of Gynaecology and Obstetrics* 59(2): 103–8.

Shea KM, Wilcox AJ, Little RE (1998) Postterm delivery: a challenge for epidemiological research. *Epidemiology* 9(2): 199–204.

Sherer DM, Spong CY, Minior VK, Salafia CM (1996) Decreased amniotic fluid volume at 32 weeks of gestation is associated with decreased fetal movements. *American Journal of Perinatology* 13(8): 479–82.

Sikorski J, Wilson J, Clement S, Das S, Smeeton N (1996) A randomised controlled trial comparing two schedules of antenatal visits: the antenatal care project. *British Medical Journal* 312(7030): 546–53.

Siney C (1994) Team effort helps pregnant drug users. *Modern Midwife* February: 23–4.

Smith DK, Shaw RW, Marteau TM (1994) Informed consent to undergo serum screening for Down's Syndrome: the gap between policy and practice. *British Medical Journal* 309(6957): 776.

Smith DK, Marteau TM. (1995) Detecting fetal abnormality: serum screening and fetal anomaly scans. *British Journal of Midwifery* 3(3): 133–6.

Smith JA, Mitchell S (1996) Debriefing after childbirth: a tool for effective risk management. *British Journal of Midwifery* 4(11): 581–6.

Smith JF, Hernandez C, Wax JR (1997) Fetal laceration injury at cesarean delivery. *Obstetrics and Gynaecology* 90(3): 344–6.

Snijders RJM, Johnson S, A Sebire NJ, Noble PL, Nicolaides KH (1996) First-trimester ultrasound screening for chromosomal defects. *Ultrasound in Obstetrics and Gynaecology* 7(3): 216–26.

Sorahan T, Hamilton L, Gardiner K, Hodgson JT, Harrington JM (1999) Maternal occupational exposure to electromagnetic fields before, during and after pregnancy in relation to risks of childhood cancers: findings from the Oxford Survey of Childhood Cancers, 1953–1981 deaths. *American Journal of Industrial Medicine* 35(4): 348–57.

Strachan DP, Cook DG (1998) Health effects of passive Smoking. 4. Parental smoking, middle ear disease and adenotonsillectomy in children. *Thorax* 53(1): 50–6.

Sratham H, Green JM, Kafestsios K (1997) Who worries that something might be wrong with the baby? A prospective study of 1072 pregnant women. *Birth* 24(4): 223–3.

Stuart JM, Healy TJG, Sutton M, Swingler GR (1989) Symphasis-fundus measurements in screening for small for dates infants: a community based study in Gloucestershire. *Journal of the Royal College of General Practitioners* 39(319): 45–8.

Symon A (1997a) Midwives and litigation: allegations of clinical error. *British Journal of Midwifery* 5(1): 70–2.

Symon A (1997b) Recollections of staff: version of the truth. *British Journal of Midwifery* 15(7): 393–4.

Symon A (1998) Causation: a medico-legal problem. *British Journal of Midwifery* 6(3): 176–9.

Thorpe-Raghdo B (1995) Newborn examinations – another delivery service. *Midirs Midwifery Digest* 5(4): 459.

Tolo KA, Little RE (1993) Occasional binges by moderate drinkers: implications for birth outcomes. *Epidemiology* 4(5): 415–20.

Tye C, Ross E, Kerry M (1988) Emergency nurse practitioner services in major accident and emergency departments. A United Kingdom postal survey. *Journal of Accident and Emergency Medicine* 15: 31–4.

UKCC (1992) *Code of Professional Conduct*. UKCC: London.

UKCC (1992) *The Scope of Professional Practice*. UKCC: London.

UKCC (1998) *Midwives Rules and Code of Practice*. UKCC: London.

UKCC (1998a) *Guidelines for Records and Record Keeping*. UKCC: London.

US Department of Health and Human Services (1990) *The Health benefits of smoking cessation: a report of the Surgeon General.* Office on Smoking and Health, Rockville Maryland. DHSS Publication No. (CDC), 90–8416.

Vio F, Salazar G, Infante C (1991) Smoking during pregnancy and lactation and its effects on breast milk. *American Journal of Clinical Nutrition* 54(6): 1011–16.

Wald NJ, Cuckle HS, Densem JW, Kennard A, Smith D (1992) Maternal serum screening for Down's syndrome; the effect of routine ultrasound scan determination of gestational age and adjustment for maternal weight. *British Journal of Obstetrics and Gynaecology* 99(2): 144–9.

Walsh RA, Redman S, Brinsmead MW, Byrne JM, Melmeth A (1997) A smoking cessation program at a public antenatal clinic. *American Journal of Public Health* 87(7): 1201–4.

Walker D (1999) Role of the routine neonatal examination (Letter). *British Medical Journal* 318(1766) (26 June).

Walkinshaw S, Pilling D, Spriggs A. (1994) Isolated choroid plexus cysts – the need for routine offer of karyotyping. *Prenatal Diagnosis* 14(8): 663–7.

Weitzman M, Gortmaker S, Klein Walker D, Sobol A (1990) Maternal smoking and childhood asthma. *Pediatrics* 85(4): 505–11.

Whittle M (1997) Ultrasonographic soft markers of fetal chromosomal defects. *British Medical Journal* 314(7085) 918.

Woollett A (1991) Having children: accounts of childless women and women with reproductive problems. In Phoenix A, Woollett A, Lloyd E (eds) *Motherhood. Meanings, Practices and Ideologies.* Sage Publications: London.

Woyton J, Agrawal P, Zimmer M (1994) Evaluation of the effect of oxytocin use for labour induction on frequency of occurrence and severity of neonatal jaundice. *Ginekol Pol* 65(12): 682–5.

Zuckerman B, Frank DA, Hingson R, Amaro H, Levenson SM, Kayne H, Parker S, Vinci R, Aboagye K, Fried LE (1989) Effects of Maternal Marijuana and cocaine use on fetal growth. *New England Journal of Medicine*, 320: 762–8.

Index